A Diagnostic Perspective on Heart Disease and Lipid Disorders

Samar K DasKundu
Libertyville, Illinois

September 12, 2017

A Diagnostic Perspective on Heart Disease and Lipid Disorders

Table of Contents

1. Introduction — 4-6
2. Lipids — 6-7
   a. Sterols — 7-12
   b. Triglycerides — 13-14
   c. Phospholipids — 14-16
   d. Sphingolipids — 16-22
3. Sphingolipidoses — 23-24
   a. Nieman Pick Disease — 24-25
   b. Fabry's Disease — 25
   c. Krabbe's Disease — 26
   d. Gaucher's Disease — 27
   e. Metachromatic Leukodystrophy — 27-29
   f. Tay-Sach's Disease — 29-30
   g. Generalized Gangliosidosis — 30-31
   h. Fucosidosis — 31-32
   i. Summary of Diagnosis and Treatment of Sphingolipidoses — 33
4. Lipoproteins — 34-41
5. Hypercholesterolemia — 42-52
6. Cardiovascular Diseases — 52-53
   a. Risk Factors — 53-58
   b. Risk Algorithm for Cardiovascular Events — 59-60
   c. Framingham Study Score — 60-61
   d. Reynold Study Score — 61-62
   e. Comparative Risk Score — 62-63
   f. Prevention — 64-65
7. LDL Particle Size and Particle Number in Cardiovascular Disease — 65-69
8. Measurement of LDL-Cholesterol — 69-72
9. Direct Measurement of LDL-Cholesterol — 72-78
10. Oxidized LDL-Cholesterol — 78-79
11. Direct Measurement of VLDL-Cholesterol — 79-88
12. Cardiac Biomarkers — 88-89
    a. Troponin — 89-90
    b. Creatine Kinase-MB — 90-92
    c. Myoglobin — 92-93
    d. Lactate Dehydrogenase — 93-94

A Diagnostic Perspective on Heart Disease and Lipid Disorders

13. Testing Strategies of Myocardial Infarction — 94-95
14. Prognostic Value of Troponin Measurement — 95-96
15. Non-Enzymatic Cardiac Biomarkers — 97
    a. Lipoprotein (a) — 97-103
    b. Homocysteine — 104-105
    c. Heart-Type Fatty Acid Binding Protein (H-FABP) — 105-108
    e. Natriuretic Peptides: BNP and NT-proBNP — 108-113
    e. C- Reactive Protein — 113-116
    f. Myeloperoxidase — 116-117
16. Conclusion — 128
17. Bibliography — 119-126
18. Dedication — 127

A Diagnostic Perspective on Heart Disease and Lipid Disorders

1. Introduction

In diagnostics Biological Marker abbreviated as Biomarker is used as a "measurable and quantifiable biological parameters (e.g., specific enzyme concentration, specific hormone concentration, specific gene phenotype distribution in a population, presence of biological substances) which serve as indices for health- and physiology-related assessments in disease conditions. The definition was improvised in 2001 by an NIH working group as "a characteristic that is objectively measured and evaluated as an indicator of normal biological processes, pathogenic processes, or pharmacologic responses to a therapeutic intervention and defined types of biomarkers.

Biomarkers can indicate a variety of health or disease characteristics, including the level or type of exposure to an environmental factor, genetic susceptibility, genetic responses to exposures, markers of subclinical or clinical disease, or indicators of response to therapy. Thus, biomarkers serve as indicators of disease trait (risk factor or risk marker), disease state (preclinical or clinical), or disease rate (progression). Accordingly, biomarkers can be classified in identifying the risk of developing an illness, screening for subclinical disease, diagnostic biomarkers, disease severity, or prognostic predicting future disease

A Diagnostic Perspective on Heart Disease and Lipid Disorders

course, including recurrence and response to therapy, and monitoring efficacy of therapy

Cardiac biomarkers are substances that are released into the blood when the heart is damaged or stressed. Measurements of these biomarkers are used to help diagnose acute coronary syndrome (ACS) and cardiac ischemia, conditions associated with insufficient blood flow to the heart.

In this book, I will review the role of various aspects of Biomarkers associated with heart disease and in lipid disorders

Cardiovascular Heart Disease (CHD) remains the leading cause of death and disability in in recent years. About 13 million Americans have CHD, 1.5 million have a myocardial infarction (MI) each year, and nearly 500,000 die of CHD each year. Although as many women as men die of CHD per year, the mean age at death from CHD is substantially higher in women. CHD is caused by atherosclerosis, a process characterized by endothelial dysfunction—in association with hypertension, diabetes, smoking, and elevated homocysteine concentrations— and cholesterol deposition in macrophages and smooth muscle cells in the arterial wall as the result of elevated LDL, lipoprotein(a), and remnant lipoproteins and decreased HDL. In addition,

A Diagnostic Perspective on Heart Disease and Lipid Disorders

smooth muscle proliferation, inflammation, and calcification occur in this process. Thrombosis, occurring after plaque rupture and aggravated by elevated fibrinogen concentrations, is often the terminal event occluding the artery. Narrowing of coronary arteries causes angina pectoris or chest pain, especially with exertion, whereas occlusion can cause MI or death of heart muscle. Blood pressure is a key factor in the development of atherosclerosis; this process does not develop on the venous side of the circulation.

2. Lipids and Lipoproteins

Lipids consists of a broad group of naturally occurring molecules that include fats, waxes, sterols including cholesterol, fat-soluble vitamins (such as vitamins A, D, E, and K), monoglycerides, diglycerides, triglycerides, phospholipids, and others. All lipids may be defined as hydrophobic or amphiphilic small molecules. The amphiphilic nature of some lipids allows them to form structures such as vesicles, liposomes, or membranes in an aqueous environment. Lipids typically do not travel alone in the blood. Instead, it binds to a protein that transports it to its destination in the body. The main biological functions of lipids include storing energy, signaling, and acting as structural components of cell membranes..

A Diagnostic Perspective on Heart Disease and Lipid Disorders

Lipids may be divided into five major categories as shown in Table 1. Although the term *lipid* is sometimes used as a synonym for fats, fats are a subgroup of lipids

Major Categories of Lipids

a. Sterols
b. Triglycerides
c. Phospholipids
d. Sphingolipids
e. Lipoproteins

a. Sterols

Sterol lipids, such as cholesterol and its derivatives, are a vital components of membrane lipids, along with the glycerophospholipids and sphingomyelins. The steroids, all derived from the same fused four-ring core structure, have different biological roles as hormones and signaling molecules. Cholesterol is a steroid alcohol found exclusively in animals and virtually in all cells and body fluids. It is precursor of variety of physiologically important steroids, including the bile acids and steroid hormones.

A Diagnostic Perspective on Heart Disease and Lipid Disorders

Cholesterol

Formula I

Cholesteryl Ester

β-Sitosterol

Cholesterol is a type of lipid molecule, and is biosynthesized by all animal cells, because it is an essential structural component of all animal cell membranes; essential to maintain both membrane structural integrity and fluidity. Cholesterol is the principal sterol synthesized by all animals and is essential for all animal life, in

A Diagnostic Perspective on Heart Disease and Lipid Disorders

vertebrates, hepatic cells typically produce the greatest amounts of cholesterol. A human male weighing 68 kg (150 lbs.) normally synthesizes about 1 gram (1,000 mg) per day, and his body contains about 35 g, mostly contained within the cell membranes. Typical daily cholesterol dietary intake for a man in the United States is 307 mg (above the upper limit recommended by the Dietary Guidelines Advisory Committee).

A human male weighing 68 kg (150 lbs.) normally synthesizes about 1 gram (1,000 mg) per day, and his body contains about 35 g, mostly contained within the cell membranes. Typical daily cholesterol dietary intake for a man in the United States is 307 mg (above the upper limit recommended by the Dietary Guidelines Advisory Committee).

Cholesterol is ingested by human are mostly esterified which is poorly absorbed. The body also compensates for any absorption of additional cholesterol by reducing cholesterol synthesis. For these reasons, cholesterol in food is digested after seven to ten hours after ingestion. However, during the first seven hours after ingestion of cholesterol is being distributed around the body within extracellular water by the various lipoproteins which transport all fats in the water outside cells causing increase

A Diagnostic Perspective on
Heart Disease and Lipid Disorders

in concentrations. Cholesterol is recycled in the body. The liver excretes it in a non-esterified form (via bile) into the digestive tract. Typically, about 50% of the excreted cholesterol is reabsorbed by the small intestine back into the bloodstream. However, sterols from plants called phytosterols (such as β-sitosterol), which can compete with cholesterol for reabsorption in the intestinal tract, thus potentially reducing cholesterol reabsorption. When intestinal lining cells absorb phytosterols, in place of cholesterol, they usually excrete the phytosterol molecules back into the gastrointestinal tract, an important protective mechanism.

Cholesterol is a major component (almost 30%) of all animal cell membranes and is required to build and maintain membranes and modulates membrane fluidity over the range of physiological temperatures. The hydroxyl group on cholesterol interacts with the polar heads of the membrane phospholipids and sphingolipids, while the bulky steroid and the hydrocarbon chain are embedded in the membrane, alongside the nonpolar fatty-acid chain of the other lipids. Through the interaction with the phospholipid fatty-acid chains, cholesterol increases membrane packing, which both alters membrane fluidity and maintains membrane integrity so that animal cells do not need to build cell walls. The membrane

A Diagnostic Perspective on Heart Disease and Lipid Disorders

remains stable and durable without being rigid, allowing animal cells to change shape and animals to move

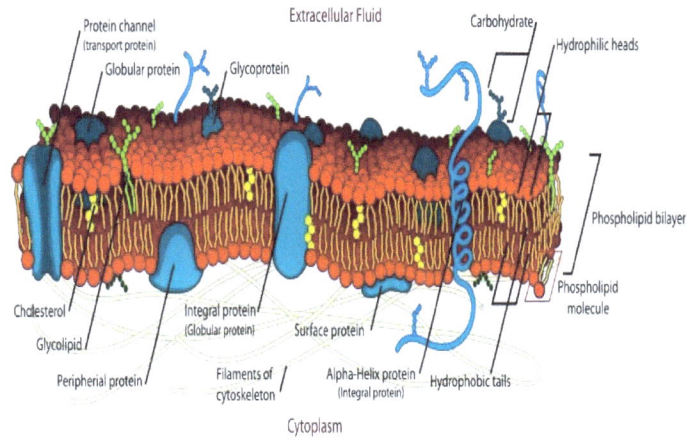

Schematic Diagram of Cell Membrane
(Image created by *LadyofHats Mariana Ruiz*)
(*Source: h*ttps://en.wikipedia.org/wiki/Cell_membrane)

The structure of the tetracyclic ring of cholesterol contributes to the fluidity of the cell membrane, as the molecule is in a *trans* conformation making all but the side chain of cholesterol rigid and planar. In this structural role, cholesterol also reduces the permeability of the plasma membrane to neutral solutes, hydrogen ions, and ions. Within the cell membrane, cholesterol also functions in intracellular transport, cell signaling and nerve conduction.

Cholesterol along with triglycerides and phospholipids are present in all animal fats in varying amounts. From a dietary

A Diagnostic Perspective on Heart Disease and Lipid Disorders

perspective, all animal fats manufacture cholesterol in varying proportions. Although phytosterols present in plant cells do compete with the cholesterol in reducing the adsorption in the intestines is not enough to have a significant impact on blocking cholesterol absorption. Phytosterols can be supplemented through the use of phytosterol-containing functional foods or dietary supplements that are recognized to reduce cholesterol levels. Some supplemental guidelines have recommended doses of phytosterols in the 1.6-3.0 grams per day range (Health Canada, EFSA, ATP III, FDA).

In 2016, the United States Department of Agriculture Dietary Guidelines Advisory Committee recommended that Americans eat as little dietary cholesterol as possible. Increased dietary intake of industrial trans fats is associated with an increased risk in all-cause mortality and cardiovascular diseases. Trans fats have been shown to reduce levels of HDL while increasing levels of LDL. Based on such evidence and evidence implicating low HDL and high LDL levels in (see Hypercholesterolemia), many health authorities advocate reducing LDL-cholesterol through changes in diet in addition to other lifestyle modifications.

A Diagnostic Perspective on Heart Disease and Lipid Disorders

b. Triglycerides

Trigycerides are esterified fatty acids with glycerol or can be non-esterified (NEFAs). Triglycerides are the main constituents of body fat in humans and other animals, as well as vegetable fat. There are diverse types of triglyceride, with the main division between saturated and unsaturated types. Plasma NEFAs liberated from adipose tissue by enzyme lipase are transported to the liver and muscle bound to albumin. Triglycerides are transported from the intestine to different tissues including liver and adipose tissue. Following hydrolysis, fatty acids are esterified and stored as triglycerides. In the human body, high levels of triglycerides in the bloodstream have been linked to atherosclerosis and, by extension, the risk of heart disease and stroke.

Structure of Triglyceride

Glycerol (left), Palmitic acid, Oleic acid, α-linolenic acid (top to bottom) (Source: https://en.wikipedia.org/wiki/Triglyceride)

A Diagnostic Perspective on Heart Disease and Lipid Disorders

The National Cholesterol Education Program has set guidelines for triglyceride levels:

Level		Interpretation
(mg/dL)	(mmol/L)	
< 150	< 1.70	Normal range – low risk
150–199	1.70–2.25	Slightly above normal
200–499	2.26–5.65	Some risk
500 or higher	> 5.65	Very high – high risk

These levels are tested after fasting 8 to 12 hours. Triglyceride levels remain temporarily higher for a period after eating.

The American Heart Association recommends an optimal triglyceride level of 100 mg/dL (1.1 mmol/L) or lower to improve heart health.

c. Phospholipids

Phospholipids are complex lipids similar in structure to triglyceride but containing phosphate and a nitrogenous base in place of one the fatty acids. They are very critical in the structural role of all membranes and the phosphate group renders the solubility on non-polar lipids and cholesterol in lipoproteins.

A Diagnostic Perspective on Heart Disease and Lipid Disorders

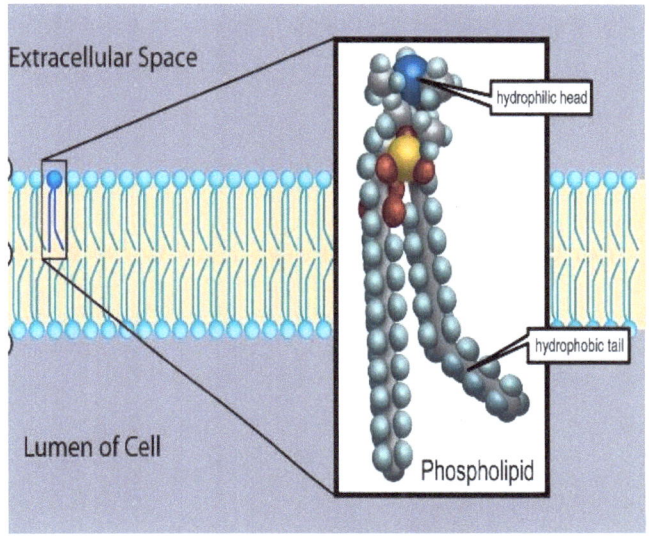

Structure of Phospholipids
(Source: https://en.wikipedia.org/wiki/Phospholipid)

The cell membrane consists of two adjacent layers of phospholipids, which form a bilayer. The fatty acid tails of phospholipids face inside, away from water, whereas the phosphate heads face the outward aqueous side. Since the heads face outward, one layer is exposed to the interior of the cell and one layer is exposed to the exterior. As the phosphate groups are polar and hydrophilic, they are attracted to water in the intracellular fluid. **The phospholipid bilayer is a universal component of all cell membranes. Its role is critical because its structural components provide the barrier that marks the boundaries of a cell. The structure is called a "lipid bilayer" because it is composed of two layers of fat cells organized in two sheets. he cell membrane is selectively permeable to ions and organic molecules and controls the movement of substances in and out of cells. The basic function of the cell membrane is to protect the cell from its surroundings.

It consists of the lipid bilayer with embedded proteins. Cell membranes are involved in a variety of cellular processes such as cell adhesion, ion conductivity and cell signaling and serve as the attachment surface for several extracellular structures, including the cell wall, glycocalyx, and intracellular cytoskeleton.

d. *Sphingolipids*

Sphingolipids or Sphingoglycolipids are a class of lipids containing a backbone of spingoid bases, a set of aliphatic amino alcohols that includes sphingosine. They were discovered in brain extracts in the 1870s and were named after the mythological Sphinx because of their enigmatic nature. These compounds play important roles in signal transmission and cell recognition. Sphingolipidoses are a class of lipid storage disorders relating to sphingolipid metabolism. The main members of this group are Niemann–Pick disease, Fabry disease, Krabbe's disease, Gaucher disease, Tay–Sachs disease and metachromatic leukodystrophy. They are generally inherited in

A Diagnostic Perspective on Heart Disease and Lipid Disorders

an autosomal recessive fashion, but notably Fabry disease is X-linked recessive. A sphingolipid with an R group consisting of a hydrogen atom only is a ceramide. Other common R groups include phosphocholine, and various sugar complexes, collectively known as glycosphingolipids.

Sphingolipids are a class of glycolipids containing the amino sphingosine. (Alternatively, they may be considered as sphingolipids with a carbohydrate attached.) They include:

1. *Glycosphingolipids*
2. *Gangliosides*

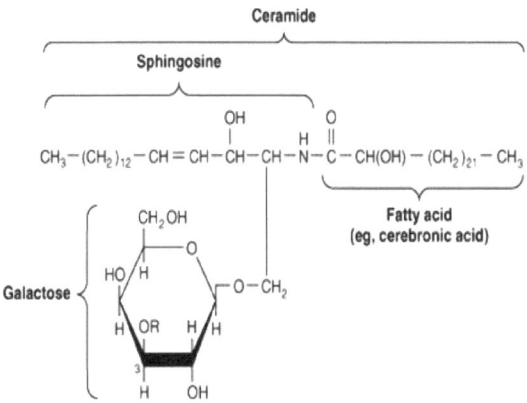

Structure of a Glycosphingolipid
(Source: http://usmle.biochemistryformedics.com/case-study-Cholera/

A Diagnostic Perspective on Heart Disease and Lipid Disorders

Subfamily series	Structure	Abbreviation
Lacto	GlcNAcβ1-3Galβ1-4GlcβCer	Lc3Cer
	Galβ1-3GlcNAcβ1-3Galβ1-4GlcβCer	Lc4Cer
Neolacto	Galβ1-4GlcNAcβ1-3Galβ1-4GlcβCer	nLc4Cer
	Galβ1-4GlcNAcβ1-3Galβ1-4GlcNAcβ1-3Galβ1-4GlcβCer	nLc6Cer
Ganglio	GalNAcβ1-4Galβ1-4GlcβCer	Gg3Cer
	Galβ1-3GalNAcβ1-4Galβ1-4GlcβCer	Gg4Cer
Globo	Galα1-4Galβ1-4GlcβCer	Gb3Cer
	GalNAcβ1-3Galα1-4Galβ1-4GlcβCer	Gb4Cer

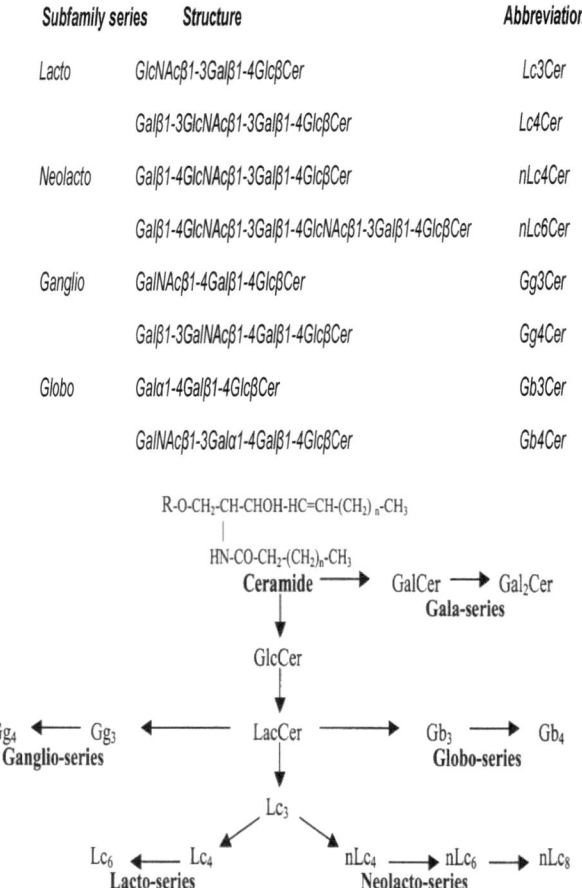

Formation of Glycosphingolipid Series from Ceramide
(Source: https://goo.gl/images/PxgUjx)

Gangliosides are the group of glycosphingolipids that show the greatest structural variation and the more complex structure. Gangliosides are characteristic of vertebrate

A Diagnostic Perspective on Heart Disease and Lipid Disorders

nervous tissues. This group includes molecules composed of ceramide linked by a glycosidic bond to an oligosaccharide chain containing hexose and N-acetylneuraminic acid (NANA or NeuNAc is an acidic sugar known also as sialic acid) units. These glycosphingolipids were discovered and named by Ernst Klenk (Z *Physiol Chemo 1942, 273, 76*) after their isolation from brain tissue. They contain sphingosine, fatty acid, hexose and neuraminic acid or sialic acid. Other investigators have since found these lipids on all cell membranes in all tissues. The heterogeneity of the brain ganglioside fraction was first shown by Svennerholm in 1956 (*Nature 1956, 177, 524*). A typical ganglioside is shown below, referred to as GM1 according to the adopted shorthand nomenclature

(*Svennerholm, Comprehensive biochemistry, viol 18, Elsevier, 1970*).

Below is recalled the structure of the most important gangliosides found in nervous tissue and other locations. The Svennerholm shorthand is used (on the right part) where G is for ganglioside, M for monosialo-, D for disialo- and T for trisialo-ganglioside. Cer, ceramide; Glc, glucose; Gal, galactose; GalNAc, N-acetyl galactosamine; NANA, sialic acid; the number 1, 2 or 3 characterizes the carbohydrate sequence. The major long-chain bases are sphingosines with 18 or 20 carbon atoms. The fatty acid is in a substantial proportion stearic acid (about 90% in the brain). The main gangliosides of the brain are GM1, GD1a, GD1b, GT1b andGQ1b present mainly outside brain tissues. Human normal cells cannot synthesize N-glycolyl-neuraminic acid, an analog of acetyl-neuraminic acid, but tumor cells do that synthesis. It has been shown that a shift from the glycolyl to the acetyl derivative may impair tumor development (*Casadesus AV et al., Glycinin J 2013, 30, 687*). There exist abnormal conditions in which genetic defects in catabolism lead to ganglioside accumulations. In generalized gangliosidosis, GM1 accumulates in the nervous system leading to mental retardation and liver enlargement. GM2 accumulation can result from inherited defects in either the hexosaminidase a or b subunit, or in the GM2 activator protein, leading to Tay-Sachs disease (B variant), Sandhoff disease (O variant), or GM2 activator deficiency (AB variant), respectively.

A Diagnostic Perspective on Heart Disease and Lipid Disorders

Ganglioside GM1(a)

Ganglioside GD1a

Ganglioside GD1b

Ganglioside GT1b

A Diagnostic Perspective on Heart Disease and Lipid Disorders

Structures of Major Brain Gangliosides

3. Sphingolipidoses

Sphingolipidoses constitutes heterogeneous group of inherited disorders of lipid metabolism affecting primarily the central nervous system. These disorders generally occur in the pediatric population. These disorders are of degenerative nature and generally characterized by diffuse and progressive involvement of neurons (gray matter) with psychomotor retardation and of fiber tracts (white matter) with weakness and spasticity. Biochemical research has identified the defects in the sphingolipidoses to specific lysosomal enzymes.

A Diagnostic Perspective on Heart Disease and Lipid Disorders

This review will cover the following:

(1) *Niemann-Pick disease lacks sphingomyelinase*

(2) *Krabbe's disease lacks galactocerebrosidase*

(3) *Gaucher's disease lacks beta-D-glucosidase*

(4) *metachromatic leukodystrophy lacks sulfatase*

(5) *Tay-Sachs disease lacks hexosaminidase A*

(6) *Fabry's disease lacking α-galactosidase*

(5) *generalized gangliosidosis lacks β-galactosidase.*

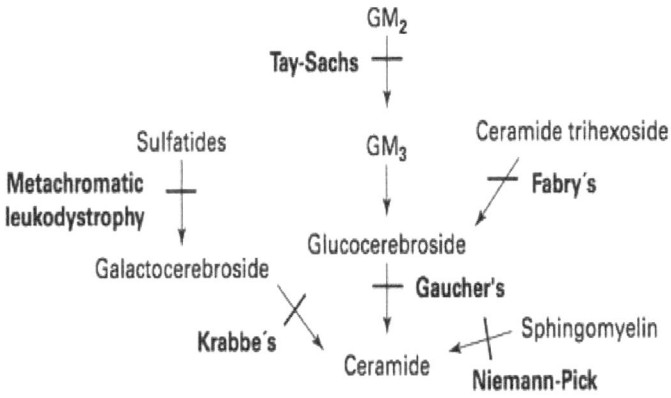

Formation of some of the Sphingolipidoses
(Source: ttps://en.wikipedia.org/wiki/Sphingolipidoses

A Diagnostic Perspective on Heart Disease and Lipid Disorders

Common Sphingolipidoses

Lyposomal Storge Disease	Enzyme deficiency	Accumulating substance
Tay-Sachs disease	Hexosaminidase A	GM2 ganglioside
Niemann-Pick disease	Sphingomyelinase	Sphingomyelin
Gaucher's disease	Glucocerebrosidase	Glucocerebroside
Fabry disease	α-Galactosidase A	Ceramide trihexoside
Metachromatic leukodystrophy	Arylsulfatase A	Sulfatides
Krabbe's disease (Globoid cell leukodystrophy)	β-Galactocerebrosidase	Galactocerebroside
Fucosidosis	Fuc-H1 and Fuc-GM1	α-Fucosidase

a. Niemann-Pick disease

Niemann-Pick disease is a genetic disorder subdivided into four groups depending upon the age of onset and clinical manifestations. The infantile form or Crocker's type A accounts for approximately 85 percent of the cases of Niemann-Pick disease and definitive lipid abnormalities in brain are limited to this subgroup. Here only this subgroup is discussed. The infantile form of Niemann-Pick disease is characterized clinically by psychomotor retardation with

A Diagnostic Perspective on Heart Disease and Lipid Disorders

mental deterioration, seizures, spasticity, hepatosplenomegaly and frequently the presence of a "cherry red spot" in the fundi. Pathological examination of enlarged visceral organs, brain and bone marrow discloses the presence of "foam cells" laden with lipid material. Analysis of the lipid reveals an abundance of sphingomyelin and lack of the hydrolytic enzyme sphingomyelinase.

b. Fabry disease

Fabry disease is a rare genetic lysosomal storage disease, inherited in an X-linked manner. Fabry disease can cause a wide range of systemic symptoms. Symptoms are typically first experienced in early childhood and can be very difficult to understand. Full body or localized pain to the extremities (known as acroparesthesia) or gastrointestinal (GI) tract is common in patients with Fabry disease. This acroparesthesia is believed to be related to the damage of peripheral nerve fibers that transmit pain. GI tract pain is likely caused by accumulation of lipids in the small vasculature of the GI tract which obstructs blood flow and causes pain. Fabry disease is suspected based on the individual's clinical presentation, and can be diagnosed by an enzyme assay of measure the level of α-galactosidase activity.

A Diagnostic Perspective on Heart Disease and Lipid Disorders

c. Krabbe's Disease

Krabbe's disease is an autosomal, recessive, genetic disorder affecting primarily the central nervous system. Following normal early development, the disease has its onset during the middle of the first year of life. This disease show symptoms of psychomotor retardation, tonic seizures, spasticity and blindness. Histological examination of brains shows diffuse demyelination of white matter with arcuate fiber sparing. In addition, there is the characteristic accumulation of large epithelioid or "globoid" cells in the white matter and called "globoid cell leukodystrophy." Lipid analyses of brains affected with Krabbe's disease indicate a higher relative concentration of galactocerebroside. A postulated enzyme defect in this disorder is unique, because it is in the synthetic as opposed to the more common catabolic pathway. The deficient enzyme is the cytoplasmic perbromide, sulfotransferase. Recent studies showed compelling evidence in human brain tissue that the metabolic defect in Krabbe's disease is in fact a catabolic enzyme, namely, the lysosomal galactocerebroside-β - galactocerebrosidase.

A Diagnostic Perspective on Heart Disease and Lipid Disorders

d. Gaucher's Disease

Gaucher's disease is an autosomal, recessive genetic disorder that has its onset in infancy or adulthood and infrequently during adolescence. The infantile form characteristically affects the central nervous system and is sometimes referred to as the "cerebral form" of Gaucher's disease. Clinically this disease is like Niemann-Pick disease similar to psychomotor retardation, poor feeding due to bulbar weakness, spasticity, and striking hepatosplenomegaly. The lipid accumulation is due to glucocerebroside. Investigations for an enzyme defect have revealed an absence of lvsosomal β-D-glucosidase, essential for the normal degradation of glucocerebrosides.

e. Metachromatic Leukodystrophy

Metachromatic leukodystrophy (MLD or sulfatide lipidosis) is an autosomal, recessive, genetic disorder that becomes manifest during childhood and occasionally in adulthood. The symptoms in childhood are those of leukodystrophy, in that motor symptoms predominate. Muscular weakness and wasting, may be the initial symptom. MLD is unique among the sphingolipidoses because the peripheral nervous system is affected. Thus, evidence of a peripheral neuropathy with sensory, motor, and reflex changes may

A Diagnostic Perspective on Heart Disease and Lipid Disorders

precede or supersede the findings of a leukodystrophy. With progression of the disease, generalized cerebral dysfunction develops. Seizures occur in one half the patients, blindness in one-third, and death follows a decerebrate or decorticate state. The adult form of MLD usually presents as an organic dementia or psychosis, frequently diagnosed as schizophrenia. Histochemical studies disclose the presence of intracellular lipids, not only in the central and peripheral nervous systems, but also within visceral organs, such as kidney, liver, and gallbladder. Impairment of these organs does not become clinically apparent. In addition to the deposition of sulfatide within white matter cells, there is symmetrical demyelination of white matter with U-fiber or arcuate fiber sparing. Austin in the United States and Jatzkewitz in Germany. Lipid analyses in MLD reveal a ten-fold increase in brain sulfatide concentration with an inversion of the sulfatide: cerebroside ratio to 4:1. Normally the ratio is approximately 0.25 to 1. Analysis of the lipid composition of myelin in MLD demonstrates a preponderance of sulfatide; this has led to the speculation that demyelination in this disease may be due to formation of an unstable membrane. Although the clinical diagnosis of MLD is suggested by the presence of leukodystrophic symptoms and signs combined with a peripheral neuropathy. A sensitive and accurate test is the

A Diagnostic Perspective on Heart Disease and Lipid Disorders

detection of arylsulfatase in urine. Affected persons have no enzyme activity. Biochemical studies on tissues from MLD have identified an absence of sulfatase, the lysosomal enzyme which hydrolyses the sulfate group from sulfatide. Clinical investigations of sulfated compound reveal a slow turnover in MLD compared to normal subjects. These findings would support in vitro biochemical data of defective catabolism of sulfatide.

f. Tay-Sachs Disease

Tay-Sachs disease or infantile amaurotic familial idiocy (AI) is a genetic disease occurring primarily in Jewish infants. The disorder commences during the middle of the first year of life after an apparently normal early development. Death ensues after a period of two to four years. The disease is involved with the central nervous system, particularly the grey matter and so-called "cherry-red spot" of the macular region is to be seen on funduscopic examination. In addition, grey matter involvement gives rise to a cortical irritative phenomenon, manifested by myoclonic seizures. Pathological examination reveals "ballooned" neurons filled with lipid staining material. Electron microscopic studies of the involved neurons disclose the cytoplasm to be filled with membranous, lamellated bodies termed "membranous cytoplasmic bodies" or MCBs. Lipid analysis of these

A Diagnostic Perspective on Heart Disease and Lipid Disorders

bodies, reveals an increase of monosialoganglioside GM2 ganglioside and is referred to as the "Tay-Sachs ganglioside". The enzymatic defect in Tay-Sachs disease is now known to be an absence of a lysosomal beta-D-N-acetylhexosaminidase. The diagnosis of Tay-Sach's disease may be possible before birth by finding a deficiency of hexosaminidase. This technique of amniocentesis holds great promise as a powerful diagnostic tool and opens doors for its utilization for antepartum diagnosis in other genetic disorders.

g. Generalized Gangliosidosis

Generalized gangliosidosis or GM1 gangliosidosis, type is an acute infantile disease characterized by psychomotor retardation, hepatosplenomegaly, and coarse features similar to those of Hurler's disease. Generalized gangliosidosis is due to an accumulation of GM1 ganglioside in brain and viscera as well as mucopolysaccharide in the latter. Death ensues in the first two years of life. The disease has been confused with Tay-Sachs disease because of the finding of a "cherry red spot in the macula and psychomotor retardation, with Hurler's disease because of the presence of similar phenotypic abnormalities. Enzymic studies disclose a pronounced deficiency of β- galactosidase which accounts for

A Diagnostic Perspective on Heart Disease and Lipid Disorders

accumulation of the GM1 ganglioside and the mucopolysaccharide. There is yet no specific form of therapy but early recognition and diagnosis is important so that accurate genetic counseling can prevent similar births.

Juvenile GM1 gangliosidosis (or GM1 gangliosidosis, type 2) has as its onset about age one and is due to the cerebral but not visceral' accumulation of GM1 ganglioside. Death ensues within three to ten years. Although β-galactosidase is also absent in this disease, it is phenotypically distinct from generalized gangliosidosis because of the absence of usual disturbances, cherry red spot of the macula and hepatosplenomegaly.

GM2-gangliosidosis, AB variant is a rare, autosomal recessive metabolic disorder that causes progressive destruction of nerve cells in the brain and spinal cord. It has a similar pathology to Sandhoff disease and Tay-Sachs disease. The three diseases are classified together as the GM2 gangliosidosis, because each disease represents a distinct molecular point of failure in the activation of the same enzyme, beta-hexosaminidase.

h. Fucosidosis

Fucosidosis is a rare genetic disorder characterized by deficiency of the enzyme alpha-L-fucosidase, which is

A Diagnostic Perspective on Heart Disease and Lipid Disorders

required to break down (metabolize) certain complex compounds (e.g., fucose-containing glycolipids or fucose-containing glycoproteins). The inability to breakdown fucose-containing compounds results in their accumulation in various tissues in the body. Fucosidosis results in progressive neurological deterioration, skin abnormalities, growth retardation, skeletal disease and coarsening of facial features. The symptoms and severity of fucosidosis are highly variable and the disorder represents a disease spectrum in which individuals with mild cases have been known to live into the third or fourth decades. Individuals with severe cases of fucosidosis can develop life-threatening complications early in childhood).

Fucosidosis is inherited as an autosomal recessive trait. Recessive genetic disorders occur when an individual inherits two copies of an abnormal gene for the same trait, one from each parent. If an individual inherits one normal gene and one gene for the disease, the person will be a carrier for the disease but usually will not show symptoms. The risk for two carrier parents to both pass the altered gene and have an affected child is 25% with each pregnancy. The risk to have a child who is a carrier like the parents is 50% with each pregnancy. The chance for a child to receive normal genes from both parents is 25%. The risk is the same for males and females.

A Diagnostic Perspective on Heart Disease and Lipid Disorders

Fucosidosis has been successfully diagnosed before birth (prenatally) using specialized tests such as chorionic villus sampling (CVS) and/or amniocentesis. During CVS, fetal tissue samples are removed and enzyme tests (assays) are performed on cultured tissue cells (fibroblasts) and/or white blood cells (leukocytes).

Summary of Diagnosis and Treatment of Sphingolipidoses

Disease	Deficient enzyme	Accumulated products	Symptoms	Inheritance	Generally accepted treatments
Niemann-Pick disease	Sphingomyelinase	Sphingomyelin in brain and RBCs	• Mental retardation • Spasticity • Seizures • Hepatosplenomegaly • Thrombocytopenia	Autosomal recessive	Limited
Fabry disease	α-galactosidase A	Glycolipids, particularly ceramide trihexoside, in brain, heart, kidney	• Ischemic infarction in affected organs • Acroparesthesia • Angiokeratomas • hypohidrosis	X-linked	Enzyme replacement therapy
Krabbe disease	Galactocerebrosidase	Glycolipids, particularly galactocerebroside, in oligodendrocytes	• Spasticity • Neurodenegeration • Blindness • Deafness	Autosomal recessive	Bone marrow transplant (high risk), enzyme replacement (less effective)
Gaucher disease	Glucocerebrosidase	Glucocerebrosides in RBCs, liver and spleen	• Hepatosplenomegaly • Pancytopenia • Bone pain	Autosomal recessive	Enzyme replacement therapy
Tay-Sachs disease	Hexosaminidase A	GM2 gangliosides in neurons	• Neurodegeneration • Developmental disability • Early death	Autosomal recessive	None
Metachromatic leukodystrophy(MLD)	Arylsulfatase A or prosaposin	Sulfatide compounds in neural tissue	Demyelination in CNS and PNS: • Mental retardation • Motor dysfunction • Ataxia • Hyporeflexia • Seizures	Autosomal recessive	Bone marrow transplant (high risk, enzyme replacement therapy (less effective)

A Diagnostic Perspective on Heart Disease and Lipid Disorders

4. Lipoprotein

A lipoprotein is a biochemical assembly whose purpose is to transport hydrophobic lipid in blood or extracellular fluid. They have a single-layer phospholipid and cholesterol outer shell, with the hydrophilic portions oriented outward toward the surrounding water and lipophilic portions of each molecule oriented inwards toward the lipids molecules within the particles. Apolipoproteins are embedded in the membrane, both stabilizing the complex and giving its functional identity determining its fate. Many enzymes, transporters, structural proteins, antigens, adhesion molecules, and toxins are lipoproteins. Examples include the plasma lipoprotein particles classified as high density lipoprotein (HDL, low density lipoprotein (LDL), intermediate density lipoprotein (IDL), very low density lipoprotein (VLDL) and Chylomicrons, according to density / size (an inverse relationship), compared with the surrounding plasma water. These complex protein capsules enable fats to be carried in all extracellular water, including the blood stream (an example of emulsification), subgroups of which are primary drivers / modulators of atherosclerosis. Apolipoproteins are embedded in the membrane, both stabilizing the complex and giving its functional identity determining its fate. Many enzymes, transporters, structural

A Diagnostic Perspective on Heart Disease and Lipid Disorders

proteins, antigens, adhesion molecules and toxins are lipoprotein. These complex protein capsules enable fats to be carried in all extracellular water, including the blood stream (an example of emulsification), subgroups of which are primary drivers / modulators of atherosclerosis.

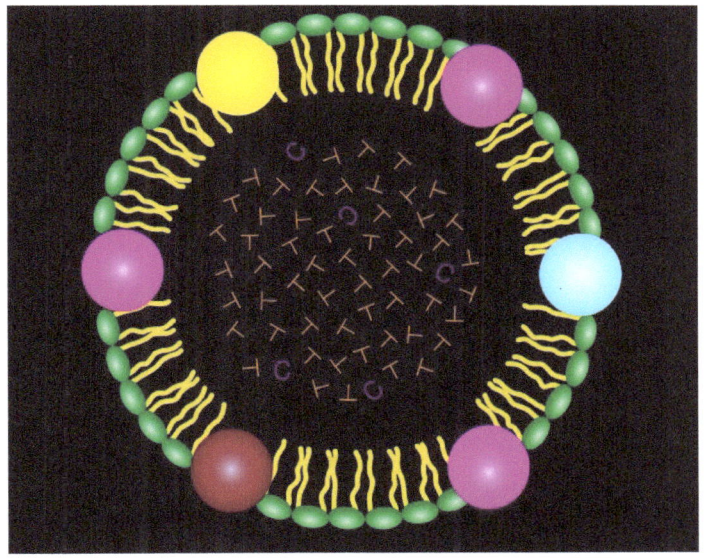

Structure of Lipoprotein Chylomicron
ApoA, ApoB, ApoC, ApoE, T (Triglyceride), C (Cholesterol);
green (Phospholipids) (Created by Usuario:Xvazquez)
(Source: https://commons.wikimedia.org/w/index.php?curid=4024624

A Diagnostic Perspective on Heart Disease and Lipid Disorders

Classification and Properties of Lipoprotein

Class	Diameter (nm)	Density (g/mL)	Source and Function	Major Apolipproteins
Chylomicrons	500	<0.95	Intestine, Transport of Dietary Triglycerides	Apo A, Apo B48, ApoC (I, II III), Apo E
Very low density liporoteins (VLDL)	43	<1.006	Liver. Transport of endogeneously synthesized Triglycerides	ApoB100, ApoC (I, II, III), ApoE
Intermediate density lipproteins (IDL)	27	1.006-1.019	Liver. Forms and stabilized Cholesterol and Triglycerides from liver to blood for transport to fatty-acid utilizing tissues	ApoE (2, 3, 4)
Low density lipoproteins (LDL)	22	I: 1.02-1.03 II: 1.03-1.04 III: 1.04-1.06	Formed in circulation by partial breakdown of Intermediate density liprotein. Delivers cholesterol to peripheral tissues	ApoB100
High density lipproteins (HDL)	8	1: 1.063-1.125 2: 1.125-1.210	Liver. Removes "used" cholesterol from tisues and takes it to liver. Donates apolipoprotens to CM and VLDL	ApoA, ApoC (I, II,III), ApoD, ApoE

Cholesterol is minimally soluble in water and so it cannot dissolve and travel in the water-based bloodstream. Instead, it is transported in the bloodstream by lipoproteins that are water-soluble and carry cholesterol and triglycerides internally. The largest lipoproteins, which primarily transport fats from the intestinal mucosa to the liver, are called chylomicrons. They carry mostly fats in the form of triglycerides. In the liver, chylomicron particles release triglycerides and some cholesterol. The liver converts unburned food metabolites into very low density lipoproteins (VLDL) and secretes them into plasma where they are converted to intermediate density

A Diagnostic Perspective on Heart Disease and Lipid Disorders

lipoproteins (IDL), which thereafter are converted to low-density lipoprotein (LDL) particles and non-esterified fatty acids, which can affect other body cells. In healthy individuals, the relatively few LDL particles are large. In contrast, large numbers of small dense LDL particles are strongly associated with the presence of atheromatous disease within the arteries. For this reason, LDL is referred to as "bad cholesterol".

High-density lipoprotein (HDL) particles transport cholesterol back to the liver for excretion, but vary considerably in their effectiveness for doing this. Having large numbers of large HDL particles correlates with better health outcomes, and hence it is commonly called "good cholesterol". In contrast, having lesser amounts of large HDL particles is independently associated with atheromatous disease progression within the arteries.

Lipoprotein particles are organized by complex **apolipoproteins**, typically 80-100 different proteins per particle, which can be recognized and bound by specific receptors on cell membranes, directing their lipid payload into specific cells and tissues currently ingesting these fat transport particles. Lipoprotein particles thus include molecular addresses which play key roles in distribution and delivery of fats around the body in the water outside cells.

Chylomicrons, the least dense cholesterol transport molecules, contain apolipoprotein B-48, apolipoprotein C,

A Diagnostic Perspective on Heart Disease and Lipid Disorders

and apolipoprotein E (the principal cholesterol carrier in the brain in their shells. Chylomicrons carry fats from the intestine to muscle and other tissues in need of fatty acids for energy or fat production. Unused cholesterol remains in more cholesterol-rich chylomicron remnants, and taken up from here to the bloodstream by the liver.

VLDL molecules are produced by the liver from triacylglycerol and cholesterol which was not used in the synthesis of bile acids. These molecules contain apolipoprotein B100 and apolipoprotein E in their shells, and are degraded by lipoprotein lipase on the blood vessel wall to IDL.

Blood vessels cleave and absorb triacylglycerol from IDL molecules, increasing the concentration of cholesterol. IDL molecules are then consumed in two processes: half is metabolized by HTGL and taken up by the LDL receptor on the liver cell surfaces, while the other half continues to lose triacyclglycerols n the bloodstream until they become LDL molecules, with the highest concentration of cholesterol within them.

LDL particles are the major blood cholesterol carriers. Each one contains approximately 1,500 molecules of cholesterol ester. LDL molecule shells contain just one molecule of apolipoprotein B100, recognized by LDL receptors in

A Diagnostic Perspective on Heart Disease and Lipid Disorders

peripheral tissues. Upon binding of apolipoprotein B100, many LDL receptors concentrate in clathrin-coated pits. Both LDL and its receptor form vesicles within a cell via endocytosis. These vesicles then fuse with a lysosome, where the lysosomal acid lipase enzyme hydrolyzes the cholesterol esters. The cholesterol can then be used for membrane biosynthesis or esterified and stored within the cell, not interfere with the cell membranes.

LDL receptors are used up during cholesterol absorption, and its synthesis is regulated by SREBP (sterol regulatory element-binding protein). In the presence of cholesterol, SREBP is bound to two other proteins: SCAP (SREBP cleavage-activating protein) and INSIG-1. The same protein that controls the synthesis of cholesterol *de novo*, according to its presence inside the cell. The cleaved SREBP that migrates to the nucleus, acts as a transcription factor to bind to the sterol regulatory element (SRE), which stimulates the transcription of many genes. Among these are the low-density lipoprotein (LDL) receptor and HMG-CoA reductase. The LDL receptor scavenges circulating LDL from the bloodstream, whereas HMG-CoA reductase leads to an increase of endogenous production of cholesterol. A large part of this signaling pathway was clarified by Dr. Michael S. Brown and Dr. Joseph L. Goldstein in the 1970s. In A cell with abundant cholesterol will have its LDL receptor synthesis

A Diagnostic Perspective on Heart Disease and Lipid Disorders

blocked, to prevent new cholesterol in LDL molecules from being taken up. Conversely, LDL receptor synthesis proceeds when a cell is deficient in cholesterol. When this process becomes unregulated, LDL molecules without receptors begin to appear in the blood. These LDL molecules are oxidized and taken up by macrophages, which become engorged and form foam cells. These foam cells often become trapped in the walls of blood vessels and contribute to atherosclerotic plaque formation. Differences in cholesterol homeostasis affect the development of early atherosclerosis (carotid intima-media thickness). These plaques are the main causes of heart attacks, strokes, and other serious medical problems, leading to the association of so-called LDL cholesterol (a lipoprotein) with "bad" cholesterol.

HDL particles are thought to transport cholesterol back to the liver, either for excretion or for other tissues that synthesize hormones, in a process known as reverse cholesterol transport (RCT). Large numbers of HDL particles correlate with better health outcomes. whereas lower amounts of HDL particles are associated with atheromatous disease progression in the arteries. The metabolism and transport of lipoproteins in blood is shown below.

A Diagnostic Perspective on Heart Disease and Lipid Disorders

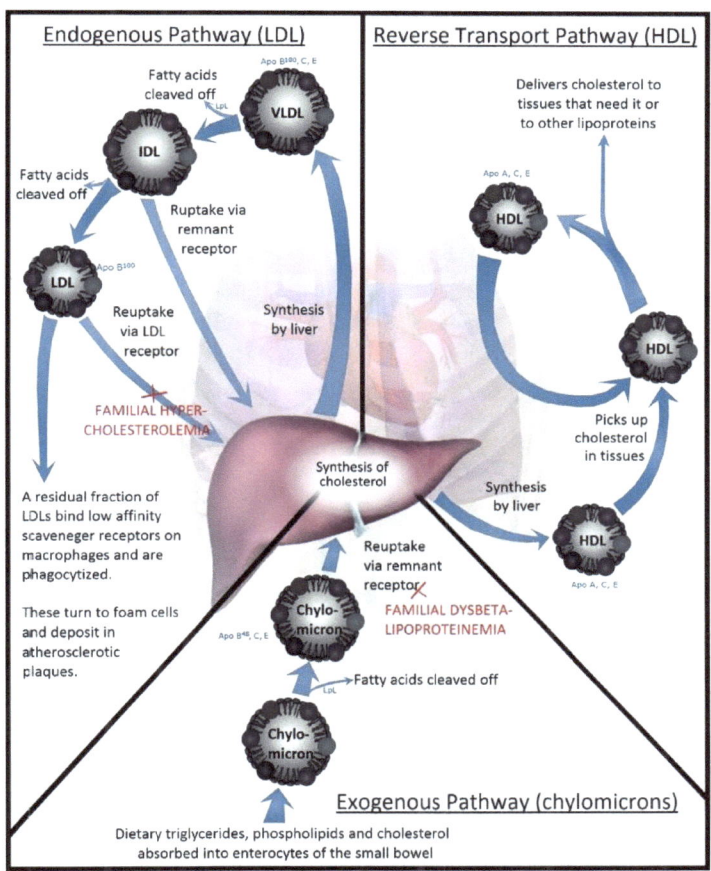

Endogenous and Exogenous Pathways of Lipoprotein Metabolism
The author thanks very much Dr. Nicholas Patchet for this diagram
(Source: https://en.wikipedia.org/wiki/Lipoprotein)

A Diagnostic Perspective on Heart Disease and Lipid Disorders

5. Hypercholesterolemia

Hypercholesterolemia, is the presence of elevated levels of cholesterol in the blood. It is a form of Lipidemia and hyperlipoproteinemia (elevated levels of lipoproteins in the blood). Hyperlipidemias are divided into primary and secondary subtypes. Primary hyperlipidemia is usually due to genetic causes (such as a mutation in a receptor protein), while secondary hyperlipidemia arises due to other underlying causes such as diabetes. Lipid and lipoprotein abnormalities are common in the general population and are regarded as modifiable risk factors for atherosclerosis and cardiovascular disease. Atherosclerosis is a specific form of arteriosclerosis in which an artery wall thickens as a result of invasion and accumulation of white blood cells (foam cells) and proliferation of intimal-smooth-muscle cell creating an atheromatous (fibrofatty) plaque. The accumulation of the white blood cells is termed "fatty streaks" early on because of the appearance being like that of marbled steak. These accumulations contain both living, active white blood cells (producing inflammation) and remnants of dead cells, including cholesterol and and triglycerides. The remnants eventually include calcium and other crystallized materials within the outermost and oldest plaque. The "fatty streaks" reduce the elasticity of the

A Diagnostic Perspective on Heart Disease and Lipid Disorders

artery walls. However, they do not affect blood flow for decades because the artery muscular wall enlarges at the locations of plaque. The wall stiffening may eventually increase pulse pressure; widened pulse pressure is one possible result of advanced disease within the major arteries.

Atherosclerosis is therefore a syndrome affecting arterial blood vessels due to a chronic inflammatory response of white blood cells in the walls of arteries. This is promoted by low-density lipoproteins (LDL, plasma proteins that carry cholesterol and triglycerides) without adequate removal of fats and cholesterol from the macrophages by functional high-density lipoproteins (HDL). It is commonly referred to as a "hardening" or furring of the arteries. It is caused by the formation of multiple atheromatous plaques within the arteries. Atherosclerosis is asymptomatic for decades because the arteries enlarge at all plaque locations, thus there is no effect on blood flow. Even most plaque ruptures do not produce symptoms until enough narrowing or closure of an artery, due to clots, occurs. Signs and symptoms only occur after severe narrowing or closure impedes blood flow to different organs enough to induce symptoms. Most of the time, patients realize that they have the disease only when they

A Diagnostic Perspective on Heart Disease and Lipid Disorders

experience other cardiovascular disorders such as stroke or heart attack. These symptoms, however, still vary depending on which artery or organ is affected. **Marked narrowing in the coronary** arteries, which are responsible for bringing oxygenated blood to the heart, can produce symptoms such as the chest pain of angina and shortness of breath, sweating, nausea, dizziness or light-headedness, breathlessness or palpitations. Abnormal heart rhythms called arrhythmias (the heart is either beating too slow or too fast) are another consequence of ischemia. Carotid arteries supply blood to the brain and neck.[1] Marked narrowing of the carotid arteries can present with symptoms such as a feeling of weakness, not being able to think straight, difficulty speaking, becoming dizzy and difficulty in walking or standing up straight, blurred vision, numbness of the face, arms, and legs, severe headache and losing consciousness. These symptoms are also related to stroke (death of brain cells). Stroke is caused by marked narrowing or closure of arteries going to the brain; lack of adequate blood supply leads to the death of the cells of the affected tissue.

Peripheral arteries, which supply blood to the legs, arms, and pelvis, also experience marked narrowing due to plaque

A Diagnostic Perspective on Heart Disease and Lipid Disorders

rupture and clots. Symptoms for the marked narrowing are numbness within the arms or legs, as well as pain.

Another significant location for the plaque formation is the renal arteries, which supply blood to the kidneys. Plaque occurrence and accumulation leads to decreased kidney blood flow and chronic kidney disease, which, like all other areas, are typically asymptomatic until late stages. According to United States data for 2004, in about 66% of men and 47% of women, the first symptom of atherosclerotic cardiovascular disease is a heart attack or sudden cardiac death (death within one hour of onset of the symptom). Cardiac stress testing, traditionally the most commonly performed non-invasive testing method for blood flow limitations, in general, detects only lumen narrowing of ≈75% or greater, although some physicians claim that nuclear stress methods can detect as little as 50%.

Atherosclerosis is initiated by inflammatory processes in the endothelial cells of the vessel wall associated with retained LDL particles. This retention may be a cause, an effect, or both, of the underlying inflammatory process. Lipoproteins in the blood vary in size. Some data suggests that small dense LDL particles are more prone to pass between the endothelial cells, going behind the cellular monolayer of endothelium. LDL particles and their content are susceptible

A Diagnostic Perspective on Heart Disease and Lipid Disorders

to oxidation by free radicals, and the risk is higher while the particles are in the wall than while in the bloodstream. However, LDL particles have a half-life of only a couple of days, and their content, namely cholesterol, phospholipids, cholesteryl esters, and triglycerides changes with time.

LDL particles can become more prone to oxidation when inside the vessel. Endothelial cells respond by attracting monocyte white blood cells, causing them to leave the blood stream, penetrate the arterial walls and transform into macrophages. The macrophages' ingestion of oxidized LDL particles triggers a cascade of immune responses which over time can produce an atheroma if HDL removal of fats from the macrophages does not keep up. The immune system's specialized white blood cells (macrophages) absorb the oxidized LDL, forming specialized foam cells. If these foam cells are not able to process the oxidized LDL and recruit HDL particles to remove the fats, they grow and eventually rupture, leaving behind cellular membrane remnants, oxidized materials, and fats (including cholesterol) in the artery wall.

This atherosclerotic disease process, over decades, leads to myocardial infarction (heart attack), stroke, and peripheral vascular disease. Since higher blood LDL, especially higher LDL particle concentrations and smaller LDL particle size, contribute to this process more than the cholesterol content of the HDL particles, LDL particles are often termed "bad

A Diagnostic Perspective on Heart Disease and Lipid Disorders

cholesterol" because they have been linked to atheroma formation. On the other hand, high concentrations of functional HDL, which can remove cholesterol from cells and atheroma, offer protection and are sometimes referred to as "good cholesterol". These balances are mostly genetically determined, but can be changed by body build, medications, food choices, and other factors. Conditions with elevated concentrations of oxidized LDL particles, especially "small dense LDL" (sdLDL) particles, are associated with atheroma formation in the walls of arteries, a condition known as atherosclerosis, which is the principal cause of coronary heart disease and other forms of cardiovascular disease. In contrast, HDL particles (especially large HDL) have been identified as a mechanism by which cholesterol and inflammatory mediators can be removed from atheroma. Increased concentrations of HDL correlate with lower rates of atheroma progressions and even regression. A 2007 study pooling data on almost 900,000 subjects in 61 cohorts demonstrated that blood total cholesterol levels have an exponential effect on cardiovascular and total mortality, with the association more pronounced in younger subjects. Still, because cardiovascular disease is relatively rare in the younger population, the impact of high cholesterol on health is still larger in older people.

A Diagnostic Perspective on Heart Disease and Lipid Disorders

Elevated levels of the lipoprotein fractions, LDL, IDL and VLDL are regarded as atherogenic (prone to cause atherosclerosis). Levels of these fractions, rather than the total cholesterol level, correlate with the extent and progress of atherosclerosis. Conversely, the total cholesterol can be within normal limits, yet be made up primarily of small LDL and small HDL particles, under which conditions atheroma growth rates would still be high. Recently, a *post adhoc* analysis of the IDEAL and the EPIC prospective studies found an association between high levels of HDL cholesterol (adjusted for apolipoprotein A-I and apolipoprotein B) and increased risk of cardiovascular disease, casting doubt on the cardioprotective role of "good cholesterol".

Elevated cholesterol levels are treated with a strict diet consisting of low saturated fat, trans fat-free, low cholesterol foods, often followed by one of various hypolipidemic agents, such as statins, fibrates, cholesterol absorption inhibitors, nicotinic acid derivatives or bile acid sequestrants. Multiple human trials using HMG-CoA reductase inhibitors, known as statins, have repeatedly confirmed that changing lipoprotein transport patterns from unhealthy to healthier patterns significantly lowers cardiovascular disease event rates, even for people with cholesterol values currently considered low for adults. Studies have also found that statins reduce

A Diagnostic Perspective on Heart Disease and Lipid Disorders

atheroma progression. As a result, people with a history of cardiovascular disease may derive benefit from statins irrespective of their cholesterol levels (total cholesterol below 5.0 mmol/L [193 mg/dL]), and in men without cardiovascular disease, there is benefit from lowering abnormally high cholesterol levels ("primary prevention"). Primary prevention in women was originally practiced only by extension of the findings in studies on men, since, in women, none of the large statin trials conducted prior to 2007 demonstrated a statistically significant reduction in overall mortality or in cardiovascular endpoints. In 2008, a large clinical trial reported that, in apparently healthy adults with increased levels of the inflammatory biomarker high-sensitivity C-reactive protein but with low initial LDL, 20 mg/day of rosuvastatin for 1.9 years resulted in a 44% reduction in the incidence of cardiovascular events and a 20% reduction in all-cause mortality; the effect was statistically significant for both genders.

The 1987 report of National Cholesterol Education Program, Adult Treatment Panels suggests the total blood cholesterol level should be: < 200 mg/dL normal blood cholesterol, 200–239 mg/dL borderline-high, > 240 mg/dL high cholesterol. The 1987 report of National Cholesterol Education Program, Adult Treatment Panels suggests the total blood

A Diagnostic Perspective on Heart Disease and Lipid Disorders

cholesterol level should be: < 200 mg/dL normal blood cholesterol, 200–239 mg/dL borderline-high, > 240 mg/dL high cholesterol.[81] The American Heart Association provides a similar set of guidelines for total (fasting) blood cholesterol levels and risk for heart disease: The American Heart Association provides a similar set of guidelines for total (fasting) blood cholesterol levels and risk for heart disease.

National Cholesterol Education Program Guideline (1987)

Cholesterol Level (mg/dL)	Cholesterol Level (mmol/L)	Interpretation
< 200	< 5.2	Desirable level corresponding to lower risk for heart disease
200–240	5.2–6.2	Borderline high risk
> 240	> 6.2	High risk

Total cholesterol is defined as the sum of HDL, LDL, and VLDL. Usually, only the total, HDL, and triglycerides are measured. For cost reasons, the VLDL is usually estimated as one-fifth of the triglycerides and the LDL is estimated using the Friedewald formula (or a variant): estimated LDL = [total cholesterol] − [total HDL] − [estimated VLDL]. VLDL can be calculated by dividing total triglycerides by five. Direct LDL measures are used when triglycerides exceed 400 mg/dL. The

A Diagnostic Perspective on Heart Disease and Lipid Disorders

estimated VLDL and LDL have more error when triglycerides are above 400 mg/dL.

However, in recent years the lipid profile is different and aside total cholesterol, LDL-cholesterol (bad cholesterol) and HDL-cholesterol (good cholesterol) and triglycerides are also measured. The following tables show the classification of Total, LDL, HDL and Triglycerides levels after 10-12 hours of fasting.

NIH ATP III Classification of Serum Total Cholesterol (mg/dL)

< 200	Desirable
200-239	Borderline High
$\geq$ 240	High

NIH ATP III Classification of Serum LDL Cholesterol (mg/dL)

<100	Optimal
100-129	Near Optimal/Above Optimal
130-159	Borderline High
160-189	High
$\geq$190	Very High

A Diagnostic Perspective on Heart Disease and Lipid Disorders

NIH ATP III Classification of Serum HDL Cholesterol (mg/dL)

< 40	Low
≥ 60	High

NIH ATP III Classification of Serum Triglycerides (mg/dL)

< 150	Normal
150-199	Borderline high
200-499	High
≥ 500	Very high

6. Cardiovascular Disease

Cardiovascular disease (CVD) is a class of diseases that involve the heart or blood vessels. They are known as vascular diseases.

- *Coronary artery disease (CAD) - this is involved in coronary heart disease and ischemic heart disease*
- *Peripheral arterial disease (PAD) – this is involved in disease of blood vessels that supply blood to the arms and legs*
- *Cerebrovascular disease – this is involved in blood vessels that supply blood to the brain (includes stroke)*
- *Renal artery stenosis- this is involved by atherosclerosis which causes the renal arteries to harden and narrow due to the build-up of plaque and affects kidney function*

A Diagnostic Perspective on Heart Disease and Lipid Disorders

The Cardiovascular diseases not involving heart are listed below:

- *Cardiomyopathy – diseases of cardiac muscle*
- *Hypertensive heart disease – diseases of the heart secondary to high blood pressure or hypertension*
- *Heart failure - a clinical syndrome caused by the inability of the heart to supply sufficient blood to the tissues to meet their metabolic requirements*
- *Pulmonary heart disease – a failure at the right side of the heart with respiratory system involvement*
- *Cardiac dysrhythmias – abnormalities of heart rhythm*
- *Inflammatory heart disease*
    - *Endocarditis – inflammation of the inner layer of the heart, the endocardium. The structures most commonly involved are the heart valves.*
    - *Inflammatory cardiomegaly*
    - *Myocarditis – inflammation of the myocardium, the muscular part of the heart.*
- *Congenital heart disease – heart structure malformations existing at birth*
- *Rheumatic heart disease – heart muscles and valves damage due to rheumatic fever*

a. Risk Factors

Coronary artery disease, stroke, and peripheral artery disease involve atherosclerosis. This may be caused by high blood pressure, smoking, diabetes, lack of exercise obesity, high blood cholesterol, poor diet, and excessive alcohol consumption, raised blood cholesterol (hyperlipidemia), psychosocial factors, poverty and low educational status, and air pollution. While the individual

A Diagnostic Perspective on Heart Disease and Lipid Disorders

contribution of each risk factor varies between different communities or ethnic groups the overall contribution of these risk factors is very consistent. Some of these risk factors, such as age, gender or family history/genetic predisposition, are immutable; however, many important cardiovascular risk factors are modifiable by lifestyle change, social change, drug treatment (for example prevention of hypertension, hyperlipidemia, and diabetes). People with obesity are at increased risk of **atherosclerosis of the coronary arteries.** Genetic factors influence the development of cardiovascular disease in men who are less than 55 years-old and in women who are less than 65 years old. Cardiovascular disease in a person's parents increases their risk by 3-fold. Multiple **single nucleotide polymorphisms (SNP) have** been found to be associated with cardiovascular disease in genetic association studies, but usually their individual influence is small, and genetic contributions to cardiovascular disease are poorly understood. Age is by far the most important risk factor in developing cardiovascular or heart diseases. Multiple explanations have been proposed to explain why age increases the risk of cardiovascular/heart diseases. One of them is related to serum cholesterol level. In most populations, the serum total cholesterol level increases as age increases. In men, this increase levels off around age

A Diagnostic Perspective on Heart Disease and Lipid Disorders

45 to 50 years. In women, the increase continues sharply until age 60 to 65 years. Aging is also associated with changes in the mechanical and structural properties of the vascular wall, which leads to the loss of arterial elasticity and reduced arterial compliance and may subsequently lead to coronary artery disease.

It is estimated that 90% of CVD is preventable. Prevention of atherosclerosis involves improving risk factors through: healthy eating, exercise, avoidance of tobacco smoke and limiting alcohol intake. Treating risk factors, such as high blood pressure, blood lipids and controlling diabetes is beneficial. Cardiovascular diseases are the leading cause of death globally. Coronary artery disease and stroke account for 80% of CVD deaths in males and 75% of CVD deaths in females. Most cardiovascular disease affects older adults. In the United States 11% of people between 20 and 40 have CVD, while 37% between 40 and 60, 71% of people between 60 and 80, and 85% of people over 80 have CVD. The average age of death from coronary artery disease in the developed world is around 80 while it is around 68 in the developing world. Disease onset is typically seven to ten years earlier in men as compared to women. Most cardiovascular disease affects older adults. In the United States 11% of people between 20 and 40 have

A Diagnostic Perspective on Heart Disease and Lipid Disorders

CVD, while 37% between 40 and 60, 71% of people between 60 and 80, and 85% of people over 80 have CVD. The average age of death from coronary artery disease in the developed world is around 80 while it is around 68 in the developing world. Disease onset is typically seven to ten years earlier in men as compared to women.

Major Risk Factors in Cardiovascular Disease:
- a. Cigarette smoking
- b. Hypertension (BP greater than or equal to 140/90 mmHg)
- c. LDL-Cholesterol ($\geq$130 mg/dL)
- d. HDL-Cholesterol (< 40 mg/dL)
- e. Triglycerides ($\geq$150 mg/dL)
- f. Fasting Glucose (($\geq$110 mg/dL)
- g. Family history of premature CHD
- h. Age (men $\geq$45 years; women $\geq$ 55 years)
- i. Obesity
- j. Excessive Alcohol consumption

A Diagnostic Perspective on Heart Disease and Lipid Disorders

The following table indicates how to control CHD using lifestyle changes (controlling diet) or taking drug therapy to reduce the LDL-Cholesterol level.

LDL- Cholesterol Goals and Cutpoints for Therapeutic Lifestyle Changes (TLC) and Drug Therapy in Different Risk Categories.

Risk Category	LDL Goal	LDL Level at Which to Initiate Therapeutic Lifestyle Changes (TLC)	LDL Level at Which to Consider Drug Therapy
CHD or CHD Risk Equivalents (10-year risk >20%)	<100 mg/dL	≥ 100 mg/dL	≥ 130 mg/dL (100-129 mg/dL: drug optional)*
2+ Risk Factors (10-year risk ≥ 20%)	<130 mg/dL	≥130 mg/dL	≥ 10-year risk 10-20%: 130 mg/dL
0-1 Risk Factor**	<160 mg/dL	≥160 mg/dL	190 mg/dL (160-189 mg/dL: LDL-lowering drug optional)

* Some authorities recommend use of LDL-lowering drugs in this category if an LDL cholesterol <100 mg/dL cannot be achieved by therapeutic lifestyle changes. Others prefer use of drugs that primarily modify triglycerides and HDL

** Almost all people with 0-1 risk factor have a 10-year risk <10%, thus 10-year risk assessment in people with 0-1 risk factor is not necessary.

A Diagnostic Perspective on Heart Disease and Lipid Disorders

Major Risk Factors of Cardiovasscular Disease including Metabolic Control

Risk Factor	Defining Level	Control Level	Needed Modification
Abdominal obesity*	Waist circumference**		
Men	>102 cm (>40 in)	≤ 39 in	Intensify Weight Management Increase Physical Activity
Women	>88 cm (>35 in)	≤ 36 in	
LDL-Cholesterol	≥ 130 mg/dL	< 130 mg/dL	MG CoA reductase inhibitors (statins) Drug Therapy
Triglycerides	≥ 150 mg/dL	≤ 150 mg/dL	Intensify Weight Management Increase Physical Activity Use Drug Therapy (Fibrate)
HDL cholesterol			Intensify Weight Management Increase Physical Activity Use Drug Thaerapy (Fibrate) or Nicotinic Acid
Men	<40 mg/dl	.> 40 mg/dl	
Women	<50 mg/dl	> 50 mg/dl	
Blood pressure	BP greater than or equal to 140/90 mmHg)	< 130/75 mmHg	Control BP using BP medicine
Fasting glucose	≥ 110 mg/dL	≥ 100 mg/dL	Control Diabetes (Type 1 and Type 2) with Medicine

* Overweight and obesity are associated with insulin resistance and the metabolic syndrome. However, the presence of abdominal obesity is more highly correlated with the metabolic risk factors than is an elevated body mass index (BMI). Therefore, the simple measure of waist circumference is recommended to identify the body weight component of the metabolic syndrome.

** Some male patients can develop multiple metabolic risk factors when the waist circumference is only marginally increased, e.g., 94-102 cm (37-39 in). Such patients may have a strong genetic contribution to insulin resistance. They should benefit from changes in life habits, similarly to men with categorical increases in waist circumference.

A Diagnostic Perspective on Heart Disease and Lipid Disorders

b. Risk Algorithms for Cardiovascular Events

The guidelines that cover the screening of patients for elevated serum lipid levels, and the treatment of patients with lipid abnormalities, mostly depends on calculations of individual patients' risk for a future cardiovascular event. The risk factors are arbitrarily divided into three major categories: nonmodifiable, modifiable, and emerging as shown in table below:

Basic Categories of Risk Factors for Future Cardiovascular Events

Category	Risk Factors
Nonmodifiable risk factors	Age, sex, family history, genetic predisposition
Modifiable risk factors	Smoking, atherogenic diet, alcohol intake, physical activity, dyslipidemias, hypertension, obesity, diabetes, metabolic syndrome, uncontrollable stress and anger
Emerging risk factors	Elevation in C-reactive protein (CRP); fibrinogen; coronary artery calcification (CAC); homocysteine; lipoprotein(a); small, dense LDL, Fatty Acid Binding Protein (FABP)

A Diagnostic Perspective on Heart Disease and Lipid Disorders

The most commonly used risk algorithms developed with United States population cohorts include the following:

- *Framingham Risk Score (FRS)*
- *Reynolds Risk Score (RRS)*
- *American College of Cardiology/American Heart Association*
- *Arteriosclerotic Cardiovascular Disease Risk Estimator (AC/AHA-ASCVD)*

c. Framingham Risk Score

The Framingham Risk Score (FRS) was developed in 1998 to assess the 10-year risk of coronary heart disease (CHD) for individuals with different combinations of risk factors. The data used was from the Framingham Heart Study, an ongoing study begun in 1948 of healthy adults. A number of revisions of the score in the Framingham of the score have been published. Notable versions include the following:

- *2002 adaption of the National Heart, Lung and Blood Institute (NHLBI) Third Report of the National Cholesterol Education Program (NCEP) Expert Panel on Detection, Evaluation, and Treatment of High Blood Cholesterol in Adults (FRS-ATP-III)*
- *2008 10-year Framingham Cardiovascular Disease (CVD risk score (FRS-CVD)*

A Diagnostic Perspective on Heart Disease and Lipid Disorders

- *2006 Lifetime Framingham CVD Risk Score (Lifetime-FRS)*
- *2009 30-year Framingham HCVD risk score (FRS-HCVD)*

The 2002 adaption added the impact of treatment for hypertension, and used only hard coronary heart disease endpoints in its calculations. The 2008 adaption included additional cardiovascular events (stroke, transient ischemic attack. The 2006 Lifetime-FRS estimates risk from age 50 based on four risk factors: total cholesterol, systolic blood pressure, cigarette smoking, and diabetes. The 2014 International Atherosclerosis Society (IAS) guidelines recommends the 2006. Lifetime-FRS for countries where recalibration values can be applied to risk calculations. The 2009 30-year FRS-HCVD estimates risk from age 45 based on a larger number of major risk factors

d. Reynolds Risk Score

The Reynolds Risk Score (RRS) was developed in 2007 with data from a 10-year study of 24,558 US women without diabetes. In addition to traditional risk factors, the algorithm also includes C-reactive protein (CRP) a biomarker for inflammation.

A Diagnostic Perspective on Heart Disease and Lipid Disorders

American College of Cardiology/American Heart Association Arteriosclerotic Cardiovascular Disease Risk Estimator. The American College of Cardiology (ACC)/American Heart Association (AHA) Arteriosclerotic Cardiovascular Disease (ASCVD) Risk Estimator, released in 2013, was designed to include participants from racially and geographically diverse cohorts, the Atherosclerosis Risk in Communities (ARIC) study, the Coronary Artery Risk Development in Young Adults (CARDIA), and the Cardiovascular Health Study (CHS). The pooled cohort equations predict the future risk of cardiovascular disease and stroke. The variables used were those used in the 10-year Framingham CVD score, but unlike the Framingham CVD, only hard disease endpoints were used in the calculation.

e. **Comparing Risk Scores**

Controversy surrounds the use of CVD risk scores as the basis for guidelines for primary prevention interventions, particularly recommendations for the management of lipid disorders and identifying patients who would benefit from pharmaceutical interventions.

Issues of accuracy of risk calculations between prediction and actual outcome (score calibration) greatly varies when the algorithms are applied to populations with differing

A Diagnostic Perspective on Heart Disease and Lipid Disorders

demographics than those of the cohort from which it was developed.

Numerous studies reported calibration disparity in risk assessment using the scores above. For example, a 2015 study utilizing data from the Multi-Ethnic Study of Atherosclerosis (MESA), measured calibration for five risk scores and found the following overestimates for the risk of cardiovascular events. Most of the scores overestimates in their prediction. This is shown below:

- *FRS-CHD: 53% in men, 48% in women*
- *FRS-CVD: 37% in men, 8% in women*
- *FRS-ATP-III: 154% in men, 46% in women*
- *ACC/AHA-ASCVD: 86% in men, 67% in women*

f. Prevention

It is predictable that up to 90% of cardiovascular disease may be preventable if established risk factors are avoided. The following are currently practiced for preventing cardiovascular disease:

- *Smoking Cessation: Reduces risk by about 35%*
- *Dietary Intervention: Reduces cardiovascular risk factors*
- *Physical Exercise: Reduces cardiovascular events by 26%*

A Diagnostic Perspective on Heart Disease and Lipid Disorders

- *Alcohol Consumption: Moderate it alcohol consumption leads to a 25–30% lower risk of cardiovascular disease. Excessive alcohol intake increases the risk of cardiovascular disease and consumption of alcohol is associated with increased risk of a cardiovascular event in the day following consumption*
- *Blood Pressure: A 10 mmHg reduction in blood pressure reduces risk by about 20%*
- *Chronic inflammatory disease like CRP*
- *Drug Therapy: Decrease non-HDL cholesterol [LDL-cholesterol, VLDL-cholesterol, and Triglycerides) with Statin and /or Fibrate treatment reduces cardiovascular mortality by about 31%*
- *Obesity: Reduction of body fat ease body fat of overweight or obese or people with severe obesity, weight loss following bariatric surgery is associated with a 46% reduction in cardiovascular risk*
- *Psychosocial stress: Mental stress–induced myocardial ischemia is associated with an increased risk of heart problems in those with previous heart disease.*
- *Chronic kidney disease*
- *Family history of premature cardiovascular disease (CVD) or familial dyslipidemia*

A Diagnostic Perspective on Heart Disease and Lipid Disorders

It is to keep in mind that most guidelines recommend combining preventive strategies. A 2015 Cochrane Review found some evidence that interventions aiming to reduce more than one cardiovascular risk factor may have favorable effects on blood pressure, body mass index and waist circumference; however, evidence was limited and it is difficult to draw firm conclusions on the effects on cardiovascular events and mortality. For adults without a known diagnosis of hypertension, diabetes, hyperlipidemia, or cardiovascular disease, routine counseling to advise them to improve their diet and increase their physical activity has not been found to be significant. Another Cochrane review suggested that simply providing people with a cardiovascular disease risk score may reduce cardiovascular disease risk factors by a small amount compared to usual care. However, there was some uncertainty as to whether providing these scores had any effect on cardiovascular disease events.

7. LDL Particle Number and Size in Cardiovascular Disease

Low density lipoprotein (LDL) is unquestionably a very powerful marker for the development of an atherosclerotic vascular event. LDL is directly involved in the atherosclerotic process and is felt to be directly toxic to the vascular

A Diagnostic Perspective on Heart Disease and Lipid Disorders

endothelium. LDL, at increased concentrations in the blood stream, enters the blood vessel wall and in the appropriate circumstances the LDL particle changes and becomes oxidized. Oxidized LDL is a major trigger of the Atherosclerotic process that ultimately culminates in plaque buildup and obstruction of the blood vessel. LDL measurements are complicated by the fact that LDL is not a single molecular species, but a multi-molecular particle aggregate composed of protein and cholesterol and other lipids. Since cholesterol is the most abundant lipid in LDL, in clinical practice LDL concentrations are routinely expressed in terms of measured or estimated cholesterol content LDL-cholesterol. What has been clear is that all people with markedly elevated LDL do not get atherosclerotic vascular disease while other individuals with modest elevations in LDL get severe disease. This can be explained by the quality of the LDL particle. Small dense LDL is more atherogenic or more toxic to the endothelium. It is more likely to enter the vessel wall, become oxidized and trigger the atherosclerotic process. Small Dense LDL is a single type of LDL another type is large buoyant LDL. Large buoyant LDL is not as toxic to the blood vessel wall and much less prone to trigger the Atherosclerosis development.

A Diagnostic Perspective on Heart Disease and Lipid Disorders

There are basically two types of assays involving blood samples to determine particle size or the presents of small dense LDL. One is the Nuclear Magnetic Resonance (NMR) particle analysis and the other is the Gradient Gel electrophoresis. Both can separate the quality and quantity of the respective types of LDL. In NMR analysis, the characteristic NMR signals broadcast by lipoprotein particles of distinct size serve as the basis for quantification of these lipoprotein subclasses in particle number concentration terms (moles of particles per liter). The concentrations of the VLDL and LDL subclasses were summed to provide total VLDL (VLDL-P) and LDL (LDL-P) particle concentrations (nmol/L). Some analyses examined the sum of LDL and VLDL particle numbers (LDL-P + VLDL-P) as a measure of total atherogenic particle concentration. Mean LDL particle size (nm diameter) was computed as the sum of the diameter of each subclass multiplied by its relative mass percentage as estimated from the amplitude of its NMR signal. Estimates of the cholesterol content of the LDL particles of individual subjects were obtained by dividing LDL-C (in mmol/L) units, obtained by multiplying the mg/dL mass concentrations by 0.0259) by LDL-P (nmol/L). This ratio provides the approximate number of cholesterol molecules per LDL particle. The observed range of values corresponds closely to those determined independently by

A Diagnostic Perspective on Heart Disease and Lipid Disorders

detailed lipid compositional analyses of isolated LDL samples of varying diameter.

Among alternative measures of LDL in this large, community-based study, LDL particle number was more strongly related to incident CVD events than LDL-C. It is of relevance to the use of specific LDL treatment targets as indicators of the adequacy of LDL lowering therapy was the finding that low LDL particle number was a better index of low CVD risk than low LDL-Cholesterol. Non-HDL-Cholesterol provided risk prediction intermediate between LDL particle number and LDL-Cholesterol, with evidence suggesting that the better prediction relative to LDL-Cholesterol was due less to non-HDL-Cholesterol including atherogenic triglyceride-rich particles (VLDL and remnants) and more to its strong correlation with LDL particle number. Finally, LDL particles are more cholesterol-depleted when LDL concentrations are lower, independent of triglycerides or LDL particle size, helps to explain why patients with low LDL-Cholesterol often have disproportionately higher numbers of LDL particles.

There are multiple therapies that can affect Small Dense LDL. The goal of therapy is to shift small dense LDL to large buoyant LDL. Lifestyle is probably the most important means of treating small dense LDL, an adequate exercise

A Diagnostic Perspective on Heart Disease and Lipid Disorders

regimen associated with a diet restricting saturated fat. Simple weight loss can affect particle composition. Treatment of diabetes is also very important in the presence of Small Dense LDL and certain anti-diabetic medications are capable of this. Cholesterol lowering drugs (Statins and Fibrates) should promote a shift in particle composition (decrease in Small Dense Particles) and in LDL-cholesterol concentrations and triglycerides to should lower atherosclerosis risks and preventing atherosclerotic events.

8. Measurement of LDL-Cholesterol

There is no reliable method for direct method for determining LDL-Cholesterol except ultracentrifugation. It is generally calculated ted by the Friedewald equation as:

[LDL-Chol] = [Total- Chol] –[HDL-Chol] - Triglycerides/5) in mg/dL

Although these assumptions may not be strictly true, the equation generally provides LDL-Chol values within a few mg/dL of those measured by the ultracentrifugation method. However, large errors in the calculated LDL-Chol concentration occur in the samples with triglycerides exceeding 400 mg/dL. In such cases, the Friedewald calculation method is unacceptable. Several studies have

A Diagnostic Perspective on Heart Disease and Lipid Disorders

been conducted in modifying Friedewald's equation so that the calculated LDL-Chol would better correlate with the ultracentrifugation method, but no significant improvement has been made. Like the ultracentrifugation method, the LDL- Chol estimated by Friedewald's equation also contains contributions from IDL Chol and Lp(a)-Chol. Despite these limitations, both methods are commonly used. Although these assumptions may not be strictly true, the equation generally provides LDL-Chol values within a few mg/dL of those measured by the ultracentrifugation method. However, large errors in the calculated LDL-Chol concentration occur in the samples with triglycerides exceeding 400 mg/dL. In such cases, the Friedewald calculation method is unacceptable. Several studies have been conducted for modifying Friedewald's equation so that the calculated LDL-Chol would better correlate with the ultracentrifugation method, but no significant improvement has been made. Like the ultracentrifugation method, the LDL- Chol estimated by Friedewald's equation also contains contributions from IDL-Chol and Lp(a)-Chol. Despite these limitations, both above methods are commonly, IDL- Chol and Lp(a)- Chol, each of which are thought to be atherogenic markers. Moreover, Lp(a)-cholesterol concentration in plasma is independent of total Cholesterol, HDL-Chol or triglycerides. Thus, the measurement of Lp(a)

A Diagnostic Perspective on Heart Disease and Lipid Disorders

should be done independently. A method for estimating Lp(a)-Chol concentration involves measuring the total Lp(a) mass in plasma [Lp(a)] and calculating the Lp(a)-Chol. Because the unfractionated plasma layer ([d >1.006 g/mL cholesterol]) also contains IDL and Lp(a) in addition to LDL and HDL, the LDL-Chol content of this fraction ([LDL-Chol) represents contributions from LDL, IDL, and Lp(a).

In the fasting state, plasma cholesterol is normally transported primarily in three major lipoprotein fractions, concentration from the total Lp(a) mass concentration. The Lp(a)-Chol concentration is assumed to be about 30% of the total Lp(a) mass concentration (Kostner et al. (1981. The calculated LDL-Chol concentration then can be corrected for Lp(a)-cholesterol using one of the following equations:

[LDL-Chol] = [Total-Chol] - [HDL-Chol] - [Triglyceride/5] - 0.3 [Lp(a)] or

[LDL-Chol] = [d>1.006 g/ml Chol] - [HDL-Chol] - 0.3 [Lp(a)]

The factor [Triglyceride/5] relates to the plasma VLDL-Chol concentration. It is assumed that all plasma triglycerides are associated with VLDL and that the ratio of 35 triglyceride concentration to cholesterol concentration associated with VLDL is about 5. Thus, the VLDL-cholesterol concentration can be calculated from the triglyceride very low-density lipoprotein (VLDL, d<1.006 g/mL), low density lipoprotein (LDL, d 1.019-1.063 g/mL) and high-density lipoprotein (HDL, d 1.063-1.21 g/mL). Lesser amounts of cholesterol are also carried out in two minor lipoprotein classes, intermediate density lipoprotein (IDL, d 1.006-1.019 g/mL) and lipoprotein (a) (Lp(a), d 1.045-1.080 g/mL). LDL is the major contributor to the plasma total cholesterol.

It is important that the Lp(a)-Chol correction be made in the LDL-Chol concentration because studies have shown that diet and drug treatment will reduce LDL-Chol levels but not Lp(a)-Chol levels and proper patient monitoring requires an accurate measurement of LDL- Chol levels. This is particularly true for patients with elevated levels of Lp(a). For example, the Lp(a) concentration in some patients have been found to be as high as 100 mg/dL. In such patients, the LDL-Chol values will be erroneous if no correction is made for Lp(a)-Chol.

9. Direct Measurement for LDL-Cholesterol

Direct methods for LDL-Chol measurement have been reported in the literature, but most of them involve selective precipitation of LDL from plasma. Three commercial kits (Boehringer Kit, Merck Kit, and Bio Merieux Kit) are

A Diagnostic Perspective on Heart Disease and Lipid Disorders

available and have been evaluated by Mulder, et al. The Boeringer Kit uses selective precipitation of LDL with polyvinyl sulfate. The cholesterol content in the supernatant is assayed and subtracted from the total serum cholesterol to obtain the LDL-Chol concentration. The Merck Kit uses selective precipitation of LDL by heparin at pH 5.12. As in the Boeringer Kit, the LDL-Chol concentration is calculated by subtraction of supernatant cholesterol from total cholesterol. The Bio Merieux Kit uses selective precipitation of LDL with polycyclic surface-active anions. After centrifugation and removal of the supernatant, the cholesterol content of the precipitate is measured. All three commercial methods agree well with isolated LDL fractions (d 1.019-1.063 g/ml) for samples with triglyceride concentrations below about 180 mg/dL but significantly overestimate the LDL-Chol concentration for samples with higher triglyceride concentrations. No direct comparison of these kits was made with the ultracentrifugation-polyanion precipitation method. Also, the presence of lipoproteins other than LDL in the precipitate was not investigated.

We have developed a Direct Method for determining LDL-Chol (**Samar Kundu:** Patent WO1993018067 A1). The present invention provides a method for determining the amount of cholesterol associated with a specific lipoprotein,

A Diagnostic Perspective on Heart Disease and Lipid Disorders

such as LDL-Chol in a sample. A lipoprotein specific binding agent (A monoclonal antibody specific for LDL prepared by the method comprising the steps of: a. immunizing a mouse or a rat with a fragment of LDL containing the T2 region of LDL or sub fragment of the T2 region of LDL, with minimum cross-reactivity with VLDL, IDL and Lp(a) from University of Berkeley, CA). In this procedure a sample are mixed with the antibody and incubated. The amount of cholesterol associated with LDL present in the sample is then determined from the amount of cholesterol present in the anti-LDL complexes formed in the reaction. Following separation of the sample and the antibody-LDL complexes, the amount of cholesterol associated with LDL in the complex is then measured. Preferably, the LDL particles are captured by a LDL specific antibody directly or indirectly bound to a solid support. This simplifies the separation of the resulting LDL-antibody complexes. Preferably, the specific lipoprotein-cholesterol particles of interest are separated from other lipoprotein cholesterol particles in the sample before the cholesterol determination is made. For example, LDL-Chol particles are selectively separated from HDL, Lp(a), IDL and VLDL-Chol particles prior to the measurement of the cholesterol associated with the LDL particles. The present method is preferred that are useful for

A Diagnostic Perspective on Heart Disease and Lipid Disorders

detecting the amount of LDL-Chol that does not VLDL, IDL and Lp(a) in a sample.

LDL-Chol measurement can also be made as follows. LDL particles present in a plasma sample are specifically captured by an LDL-specific monoclonal antibody immobilized on a solid support. After separating the solid support from the other unbound plasma lipoproteins, the cholesterol content of the bound LDL particles is estimated by releasing the cholesterol and its esters with a detergent solution. A Standard Cholesterol assay reagent comprising of cholesterol ester hydrolase, cholesterol oxidase and horseradish peroxidase is added. The liberated hydrogen peroxide is then quantitated using a Tinder dye reagent comprising of 4-aminoantipyrine and 3,5- dichloro-2-hydroxybenzenesulfonic acid. The cholesterol concentration in a sample is quantitated based on the color generation. Alternatively, a sandwich immunoassay method for the quantitation of LDL-Chol in a plasma sample can be used. This involves the specific capture of the LDL particles in the plasma sample by the LDL-specific antibody immobilized on the solid support followed by quantitation of cholesterol in the captured LDL particles by a cholesterol binding agent which is coupled directly or indirectly to a label. The LDL-Chol bound cholesterol binding agent is then

A Diagnostic Perspective on Heart Disease and Lipid Disorders

quantitated by detection and measurement of the label. Another alternative is based on an immunochromatographic assay format, in which the lipoprotein particles in the test sample bind to a labeled cholesterol binding agent. The resulting complexes then travel along a test strip by capillary action. The labeled LDL complexes are then captured by a high affinity anti-LDL specific antibody immobilized on the test strip followed by detection and measurement of the captured labeled LDL complexes.

Cholesterol binding agents bind specifically to cholesterol and include digitonin, tomatine, filipin, amphotericin B and specific binding proteins such as polyclonal and monoclonal antibodies and other synthetic and recombinant proteins that specifically bind cholesterol, cholesterol esters and/or the cholesterol associated with lipoprotein particles. Digitonin, tomatine, amphotericin B and antibodies can be used in the quantitation of cholesterol and its esters in lipoprotein particles. Digitonin and tomatine were chemically modified and then conjugated to horseradish peroxidase (HRPO) and alkaline phosphatase (AP).

The following is an illustration for Direct Measurement of LDL-Chol in a Sandwich ELSA format. The method involves incubating the sample with a solid phase having an LDL

A Diagnostic Perspective on Heart Disease and Lipid Disorders

specific binding agent, such as the LDL-specific monoclonal antibody 4B5.6 (University of Berkeley, CA), immobilized on a solid phase and the remaining non-specific binding sites of the solid phase blocked, such as with bovine serum albumin or alkali-treated casein. LDL particles are captured by the antibody on the solid phase. Digitonin or tomatine enzyme conjugates are then incubated with the solid phase. The conjugate binds to the cholesterol associated with the LDL particles on the solid phase. The quantity or presence of enzyme bound to the solid phase or the quantity of unbound conjugate remaining after incubation with the solid phase is determined by incubation of enzyme substrate with the solid phase or the solution containing unbound conjugate. The presence of cholesterol associated with the captured LDL particles is then determined from the presence of enzyme associated with the solid phase or a reduction of enzyme activity in the solution containing unbound conjugate as compared with the original conjugate solution added to the solid phase. The quantity of cholesterol associated with the captured LDL particles is proportional to the quantity of enzyme associated with the solid phase or inversely proportional to the quantity of unbound conjugate. This method is also applicable for any of the other lipoprotein particles or mixtures thereof by substituting the appropriate lipoprotein specific binding agent for the LDL specific binding agent.

10. Oxidized LDL-Cholesterol

Oxidized LDL (Ox-LDL) are known to promote atherogenesis through foam cell formation and inflammatory responses. The process involves receptor-mediated endocytosis of Ox-LDL which leads to lipid accumulation and vascular cell dysfunction including induction of apoptosis which represents major cause of plaque growth and rupture. The oxidation of LDL-Chol is one of the first steps in the development of atherosclerosis. Briefly, LDL-Chol enters the artery wall where it becomes oxidized. Ox-LDL is then recognized by scavenger receptors on the macrophages which engulf Ox-LDL, resulting in foam cell formation, vascular inflammation and the initiation of atherosclerosis. The oxidation hypothesis of atherosclerosis suggests that oxidative modification of LDL plays a crucial role and that oxidized LDL (Ox-LDL) promotes the immune and inflammatory reactions that characterize atherosclerosis. Because of its complex composition, the LDL particle is very sensitive to oxidized damage. Each LDL particle contains approximately 700 molecules of phospholipids, 600 molecules of free cholesterol, 1600 molecules of cholesterol esters, 185

A Diagnostic Perspective on Heart Disease and Lipid Disorders

molecules of triglycerides, and one molecule of apoB. Both the protein and lipid moieties can undergo oxidative modification which is a very complex biochemical process. Recent findings suggest that Ox-LDL begins to deposit in human coronary arteries before plaque formation and increasingly deposits with plaque growth. Plasma concentration of Ox-LDL seems to be associated with the risk of acute CAD events and was suggested that plasma Ox-LDL was the strongest predictor of CAD events compared with a conventional lipoprotein profile and other traditional risk factors for CAD. In summary, the oxidative modification hypothesis of atherosclerosis additional proofs is still needed.

11. Direct Measurement of VLDL-Cholesterol

Very low-density lipoprotein (VLDL) constitutes one of the major plasma lipoproteins. VLDL particles are synthesized in the liver and are involved in triglyceride metabolism and transport of these lipids from the liver. The end products of VLDL catabolism are low density lipoproteins (LDL), another major class of lipoprotein particles in plasma.

It has been suggested that disturbances in the metabolism of apoB containing lipoproteins such as VLDL and LDL correlate with incidences of. Furthermore, an increase in

A Diagnostic Perspective on Heart Disease and Lipid Disorders

VLDL levels has been associated with hypertriglyceridemia, hyperlipidemia or familial combined hyperlipidemia. Hyperglyceridemia also has been shown to correlate with an increased incidence of coronary heart disease. Many patients with hyperglyceridemia have very low levels of high density lipoprotein (HDL), another major lipoprotein in plasma. It is recommended to treat patients with coronary heart disease who concurrently have hypertriglyceridemia and low levels of HDL with drugs and pharmacologic reagents, even when these patients have acceptable levels of total and LDL-Chol.

Two methods are presently used for the quantitation of VLDL, both of which involve the measurement of VLDL-Chol. The first method uses the factor triglyceride/5 as VLDL-Chol concentration according to Friedewald equation. In this method, it is assumed that all plasma triglycerides are associated with VLDL and chylomicrons and that other VLDL remnants are not present. Chylomicrons are microscopic lipid particles that appear in the blood transiently after a fat-containing meal, are rich in triglycerides and usually have no significant effect on the total-cholesterol concentration. Although these assumptions are not strictly true, the factor triglyceride/5 usually provides good measure of VLDL-Chol when the

A Diagnostic Perspective on Heart Disease and Lipid Disorders

subject is fasting and the triglyceride concentrations do not exceed 400 mg/dL.

The second method for quantitating VLDL uses ultracentrifugation. In this method, an aliquot of plasma is used to measure the total cholesterol concentration in the sample. A second aliquot of plasma is centrifuged (105,000x g) at a plasma density concentration of 1.006 g/mL for 18 hours at 4 ^{0} C. After centrifugation, the upper layer containing VLDL is quantitatively removed and the cholesterol concentration in the isolated VLDL is measured. Alternatively, an aliquot of the remaining bottom layer, which does not contain VLDL, is used to measure the cholesterol concentration ([d>1.006 g/mL Chol]). The cholesterol concentration of VLDL (VLDL-Chol) is then calculated using the following equation:

[VLDL-Chol] = [Total-Chol]—[d>1.006 g/mL Chol]

Both methodologies suffer from a variety of problems. For example, the use of the factor triglyceride/5 is unacceptable in cases where a subject is not fasting, or where triglyceride concentrations exceed 400 mg/dL. Moreover, this method should not be used for Type III hyperlipoproteinemic patients that contain floating β-VLDL. Although several studies have been conducted to determine better ways to measure

A Diagnostic Perspective on Heart Disease and Lipid Disorders

VLDL-Chol concentrations, no significant improvement has yet been made.

The problem with the ultracentrifugation method of VLDL-Chol quantitation is that it is both time consuming and expensive to perform. Furthermore, since the method requires specialized equipment, facilities and laboratory skills, it is not suitable for routine analysis of patient samples. To complicate these matters, no alternative methodologies for measuring VLDL, such as assays which measure apoB associated with VLDL, are currently available, either for analysis of patient samples or for research purposes. Thus, there is a need for rapid, easily performed, accurate and cost-effective methods for quantitating VLDL.

Another object of this invention is to develop a method of directly measuring apolipoprotein B-100 (apoB) and cholesterol associated with VLDL from plasma easily, cheaply, quickly and accurately without the need of highly trained technicians or expensive equipment such as ultracentrifuges.

We have developed a Direct Method for determining apolipoprotein B-100 (apoB) and cholesterol associated with VLDL from plasma easily, cheaply, quickly and accurately without the need of highly trained technicians or

A Diagnostic Perspective on Heart Disease and Lipid Disorders

expensive equipment such as ultracentrifuges (Samar Kundu: US Patent 2003/0124743 Al). This procedure provides a method for determining the amount of cholesterol associated with a specific lipoprotein, such as VLDL-Chol in a sample. A lipoprotein specific binding agent (A monoclonal antibody specific for VLDL prepared by the method comprising the steps of: steps of: (a) immunizing a mouse or a rat with Apo CIII; (b) making a suspension of the mouse or rat spleen cells; (c) fusing the spleen cells with mouse or rat myeloma cells in the presence of a fusion promoter; (d) culturing the fused cells; (e) determining the presence of anti-VLDL antibody in the culture media; (f) cloning a hybridoma producing an antibody with cross-reactivity of less than 8% of VLDL, IDL,, HDL and Lp(a). A sample are mixed with the antibody and incubated. The amount of cholesterol associated with VLDL present in the sample is then determined from the amount of cholesterol present in the anti-VLDL complexes formed in the reaction. Following separation of the sample and the antibody-VLDL complexes, the amount of cholesterol associated with VLDL in the complex is then measured. Preferably, the VLDL particles are captured by a VLDL specific antibody directly or indirectly bound to a solid support. This simplifies the separation of the resulting VLDL-antibody complexes. Preferably, the specific VLDL-Chol particles of interest are

A Diagnostic Perspective on
Heart Disease and Lipid Disorders

separated from other lipoprotein cholesterol particles in the sample before the cholesterol determination is made. For example, VLDL-Chol particles are selectively separated from HDL, Lp(a), IDL and VLDL-Chol particles prior to the measurement of the cholesterol associated with the VLDL particles. The present method is preferred that are useful for detecting the amount of VLDL-Chol that does not VLDL, IDL and Lp(a) in a sample.

VLDL-Chol measurement can be made as follows. VLDL particles present in a plasma sample are specifically captured by an VLDL-specific monoclonal antibody immobilized on a solid support. After separating the solid support from the other unbound plasma lipoproteins, the cholesterol content of the bound VLDL particles is estimated by releasing the cholesterol and its esters with a detergent solution. A Standard Cholesterol assay reagent comprising of cholesterol ester hydrolase, cholesterol oxidase and horseradish peroxidase is added. The liberated hydrogen peroxide is then quantitated using a Tinder dye reagent comprising of 4-aminoantipyrine and 3,5- dichloro-2-hydroxybenzenesulfonic acid. The cholesterol concentration in a sample is quantitated based on the color generation. Alternatively, a sandwich immunoassay method for the quantitation of VLDL-cholesterol in a plasma sample

A Diagnostic Perspective on Heart Disease and Lipid Disorders

can be used. This involves the specific capture of the VLDL particles in the plasma sample by the VLDL-specific antibody immobilized on the solid support followed by quantitation of cholesterol in the captured VLDL particles by a cholesterol binding agent which is coupled directly or indirectly to a label. The VLDL-Chol bound cholesterol binding agent is then quantitated by detection and measurement of the label. Another alternative is based on an immunochromatographic assay format, in which the lipoprotein particles in the test sample bind to a labeled cholesterol binding agent. The resulting complexes then travel along a test strip by capillary action. The labeled VLDL complexes are then captured by a high affinity anti-VLDL specific antibody immobilized on the test strip followed by detection and measurement of the captured labeled VLDL complexes.

Cholesterol binding agents bind specifically to cholesterol and include digitonin, tomatine, filipin, amphotericin B and specific binding proteins such as polyclonal and monoclonal antibodies and other synthetic and recombinant proteins that specifically bind cholesterol, cholesterol esters and/or the cholesterol associated with lipoprotein particles. Digitonin, tomatine, amphotericin B and antibodies can be used in the quantitation of cholesterol and its esters in

A Diagnostic Perspective on Heart Disease and Lipid Disorders

lipoprotein particles. Digitonin and tomatine were chemically modified and then conjugated to horseradish peroxidase (HRPO) and alkaline phosphatase (AP).

The following is an illustration for Direct Measurement of VLDL-Cholesterol in a Sandwich ELSA format. The method involves incubating the sample with a solid phase having an VLDL specific binding agent, such as the VLDL-specific monoclonal antibody immobilized on a solid phase and the remaining non-specific binding sites of the solid phase blocked, such as with bovine serum albumin or alkali-treated casein. VLDL particles are captured by the antibody on the solid phase. Digitonin or tomatine enzyme conjugates are then incubated with the solid phase. The conjugate binds to the cholesterol associated with the VLDL particles on the solid phase. The quantity or presence of enzyme bound to the solid phase or the quantity of unbound conjugate remaining after incubation with the solid phase is determined by incubation of enzyme substrate with the solid phase or the solution containing unbound conjugate. The presence of cholesterol associated with the captured VLDL particles is then determined from the presence of enzyme associated with the solid phase or a reduction of enzyme activity in the solution containing unbound conjugate as compared with the original conjugate solution added to the solid phase. The quantity of cholesterol associated with the captured VLDL particles is proportional to the quantity of enzyme associated with the solid phase or inversely proportional to the quantity of unbound conjugate. This method is also applicable for any of the other lipoprotein particles or mixtures thereof by substituting the appropriate lipoprotein specific binding agent for the LDL specific binding agent.

The correlation between the present method with ultracentrifugation method with human plasma samples is shown in Figure below:

A Diagnostic Perspective on Heart Disease and Lipid Disorders

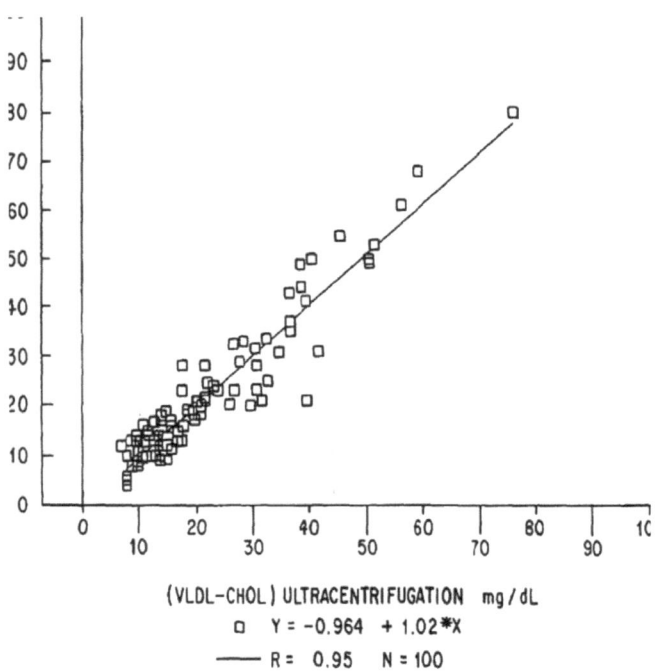

(VLDL-CHOL) ULTRACENTRIFUGATION mg/dL
Y = -0.964 + 1.02*X
R = 0.95 N = 100

12. Cardiac Biomarkers

Cardiac markers are biomarkers are used to evaluate heart function. They are often discussed in the context of myocardial infarction, but other conditions can lead to an elevation in cardiac marker level. Measuring cardiac biomarkers can be a step toward making a diagnosis for a condition. Whereas cardiac imaging often confirms a diagnosis, simpler and less expensive cardiac biomarker measurements can advise a physician whether more complicated or invasive procedures are warranted. In

A Diagnostic Perspective on Heart Disease and Lipid Disorders

variety of cases medical societies advise doctors to make biomarker measurements an initial testing strategy especially for patients at low risk of cardiac death. In earlier days, most of the cardiac biomarkers were enzymes, such as Troponins, Creatine Kinase and Myoglobin.

a. Troponin

Cardiac markers are used in the diagnosis and risk stratification of patients with chest pain and suspected acute coronary syndrome (ACS). Recently, cardiac troponins have become the cardiac markers of choice for patients with ACS. For acute myocardial infarction (MI), the consensus guidelines from the European Society of Cardiology (ESC) and the American College of Cardiology (ACC) suggest using cardiac troponin for diagnosis. The guidelines recommend that cardiac biomarkers should be measured at presentation in patients with suspected MI, and that the only biomarker that is recommended to be used for the diagnosis of acute MI due to its superior sensitivity and accuracy. Troponin is released during MI from the cytosolic pool of the myocytes. Its subsequent release is prolonged with degradation of actin and myosin filaments. Isoforms of the protein, T and I, are specific to myocardium. Differential diagnosis of troponin elevation includes acute infarction, severe pulmonary embolism causing acute right heart

A Diagnostic Perspective on Heart Disease and Lipid Disorders

overload, heart failure, myocarditis. Troponins can also calculate infarct size but the peak must be measured in the 3rd day. After myocyte injury, troponin is released in 2–4 hours and persists for up to 7 days.

The troponins are regulatory proteins found in skeletal and cardiac muscle. Three subunits have been identified: troponin I (cTnI), troponin T (cTnT), and troponin C (cTnC). The genes that encode for the skeletal and cardiac isoforms of cTnC are identical and there is no structural difference exists between them. However, the skeletal and cardiac isoforms for cTnI and troponin cTnT are distinct, and immunoassays have been designed to differentiate between them.

Two different reference ranges are used in troponin assays. The upper percentile reference limit gives the upper limit of what can be expected in a normal, healthy, adult population, while the coefficient of variation (CV) is the percent variation in assay results that can be expected when the same sample is repeatedly analyzed.

b. Creatine Kinase- MB

Creatine kinase (CK) is an enzyme expressed by various tissues and cell types. CK catalyzes the conversion of creatine and utilizes adenosine triphosphate (ATP) to

A Diagnostic Perspective on Heart Disease and Lipid Disorders

create phosphocreatine (PCr) and adenosine diphosphate (ADP. In cells, the "cytosolic" CK enzymes consist of two subunits, which can be either *B* (brain type) or *M* (muscle type). There are, therefore, three different isoenzymes: CK-MM, CK-BB and CK-MB. The primary source of CKMB is myocardium, although it is also found in skeletal muscle. CKMB levels increase with myocardial damage. Creatine kinase MB (CKMB) levels can be detected within 3 to 8 hours of the onset of chest pain, peak within 12 to 24 hours, and usually return to baseline levels within 24 to 48 hours. CK-MB test is useful if the initial troponin determination is abnormal or if a hospitalized patient has a suspected reinfarction. Prior to the introduction of cardiac troponins, the biochemical marker of choice for the diagnosis of acute MI was the CK-MB isoenzyme. The criterion most commonly used for the diagnosis of acute MI was 2 serial elevations above the diagnostic cutoff level or a single result more than twice the upper limit of normal. Although CK-MB is more concentrated in the myocardium, it also exists in skeletal muscle and false-positive elevations occur in a number of clinical settings, including trauma, heavy exertion, and myopathy.

CK-MB first appears 4-6 hours after symptom onset, peaks at 24 hours, and returns to normal in 48-72 hours. Its value in the early and late (>72 h) diagnosis of acute MI is limited.

A Diagnostic Perspective on Heart Disease and Lipid Disorders

However, its release kinetics can assist in diagnosing reinfarction if levels rise after ally declining following acute MI. See Plot below to see a comparison of Troponin and CK-MB.

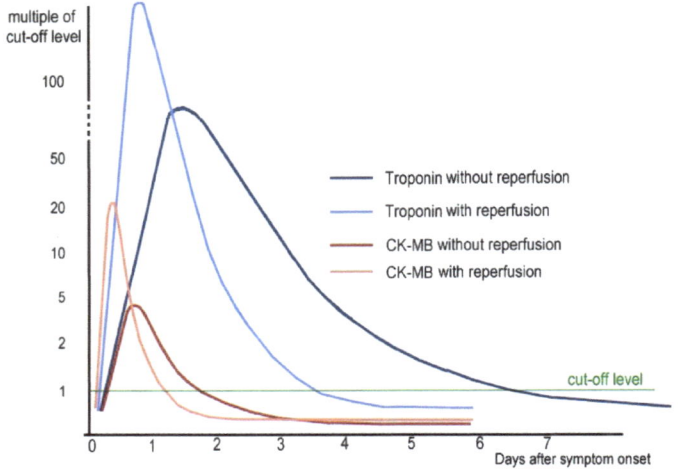

Kinetics of Troponin and CK-MB with or without reperfusion

(The author acknowledges and thanks J. Heuser for using this plot modified from ACC/AHA Practice Guidelines 2005)

c. Myoglobin

Myoglobin is a heme protein found in skeletal and cardiac muscle that was used as an early marker of MI. It has a low molecular weight and releases in 2-4 hours after onset of infarction, peaks at 6-12 hours, and returns to normal within 24-36 hours.

A Diagnostic Perspective on Heart Disease and Lipid Disorders

Rapid myoglobin assays are available, but overall, they have lack of specificity. Serial sampling every 1-2 hours can increase the sensitivity and specificity; a rise of 25-40% over 1-2 hours is strongly suggestive of acute MI. However, in most studies, myoglobin only achieved 90% sensitivity for acute MI, so the negative predictive value of myoglobin is not high enough to exclude the diagnosis of acute MI.

The original studies that evaluated myoglobin used the WHO definition of acute MI that was based on a CK-MB standard. With the adoption of a troponin standard for acute MI in the ACC/ESC definition, the sensitivity of myoglobin for acute MI is substantially reduced. This significantly diminishes its utility, and a few studies have indicated that contemporary cardiac troponin assays render the use of myoglobin measurements unnecessary.

d. Lactate Dehydrogenase

Lactate Dehydrogenase (LDH) test is a non-specific test that may be used in the evaluation of several diseases and conditions. LD is an enzyme that is found in almost all of the body's cells (as well as in bacteria) and is released from cells into the fluid portion of blood (serum or plasma) when cells are damaged or destroyed. Thus, the blood level of LDH is a general indicator of tissue and cellular damage.

A Diagnostic Perspective on Heart Disease and Lipid Disorders

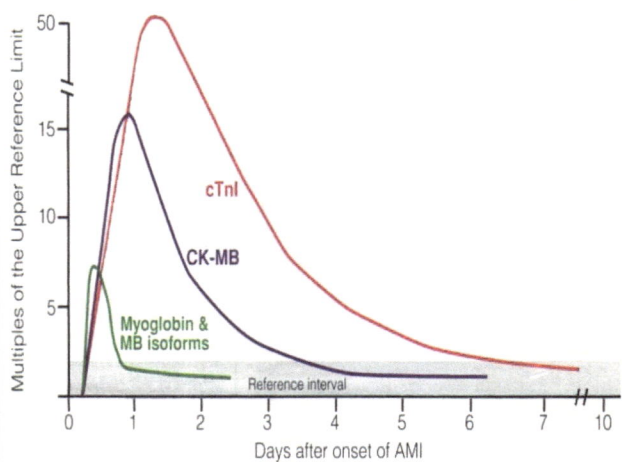

A Comparison Plot of cTnI, CK-MB and Myoglobin after the onset Acute Myocardial Infraction
(The author thanks Clarke Halfman, Ph.D. for this plot from his Lecture Series)

13. Testing Strategy for Myocardial Infarction

In patients with definite or possible ACS, serial evaluation of cardiac markers is essential to diagnosing acute MI.

1. The American College of Emergency Physicians (ACEP) recommends 3 different testing strategies for ruling out Non-ST-elevation Myocardial Infarction (NSTEMI) in the Emergency Department One strategy is to use a single negative CK-MB, cTnI, or cTnT measured 8-12 hours after symptom onset.

A Diagnostic Perspective on Heart Disease and Lipid Disorders

2. Another strategy is to use negative myoglobin in conjunction with a negative CK-MB mass or negative cTnI measured at baseline and at 90 minutes in patients presenting less than 8 hours after symptom onset.
3. A third approach is to use a negative 2-hour delta CK-MB in conjunction with a negative 2-hour delta cTnI in patients presenting less than 8 hours after symptom onset.
4. ACEP recommended a 90-minute rule-out with myoglobin was based on a study that used myoglobin in conjunction with either CK-MB or TnI. The CK-MB/myoglobin protocol yielded a sensitivity of 92% at 90 minutes, and the myoglobin/TnI combination yielded a sensitivity of 97% at 90 minutes.

14. Prognostic Value of Troponin

Troponin is generally used in the diagnosis of MI. In addition to MI diagnosis, an elevated troponin level can identify patients at substantial risk for adverse cardiac events. Specifically, data from a meta-analysis indicated that an elevated troponin level in patients without ST-segment elevation is associated with a nearly 4-fold increase in the cardiac mortality rate. In patients without

A Diagnostic Perspective on Heart Disease and Lipid Disorders

ST-segment elevation who were being considered for thrombolytic therapy, initial cTnI levels on admission correlated with mortality at 6 weeks, but CK-MB levels were not predictive of adverse cardiac events and had no prognostic value.

Other studies revealed that an elevated troponin level at baseline was an independent predictor of mortality, even in patients with chest pain and acute MI with ST-segment elevation who were eligible for reperfusion therapy.

Data from the Acute Decompensated Heart Failure National Registry (ADHERE) involving information from patients hospitalized with acute heart failure showed that increased levels of troponin and creatinine were the strongest predictors of in-hospital worsening heart failure. A number of studies demonstrated a direct correlation between the level of cTnI or cTnT and the mortality rate and adverse cardiac event rate in ACS.

A Diagnostic Perspective on Heart Disease and Lipid Disorders

15. Non-Enzymatic Cardiac Biomarkers

We describe here potential cardiac biomarkers that are not enzymes. All these markers have their own characteristics.

a. Lipoprotein(a) [Lp(a)]

Lipoprotein(a) [Lp(a)] is a genetic variant of low density lipoprotein (LDL). Although Lp(a) resembles LDL in having similar lipid composition and a common apolipoprotein B-100 (apo B), Lp(a) contains an additional glycoprotein, named apolipoprotein(a) [apo(a)]. Each Lp(a) molecule contains one molecule of apo(a) per one molecule of apo B covalently linked by a sulfide bond that can be easily reduced to LDL and apo(a) Lipoprotein(a) particles exhibit considerable inter- and intra-individual heterogeneity, with some individuals exhibiting two or more distinct Lp(a) particles differing in hydrated density. Also, the Lp(a) particle varies widely in size, with the size heterogeneity related primarily to the size of the apo(a) isoforms, 34 different isoforms have been identified. The number of apo(a) isoforms that can be distinguished varies from six to at least twelve isoforms. The smaller isoforms are generally present at less frequency and are associated with the higher Lp(a) concentrations, whereas the larger isoforms have a higher frequency and are associated with lower Lp(a)

A Diagnostic Perspective on Heart Disease and Lipid Disorders

concentrations. Apo(a) contains two types of plasminogen-like domains: a single Kringle 5 domain, with 82% amino acid sequence homology and 91% nucleotide sequence homology with plasminogen, and multiple repeats of a Kringle 4 domain, with 61-75% amino acid homology and 75-85% nucleotide sequence homology with the Kringle 4 domain of plasminogen. Numerous studies have indicated that elevated levels of Lp(a) in plasma are associated with premature coronary heart disease (CHD) Lp(a) concentrations in human plasma range from 1 mg/dL to more than 100 mg/dL. When the plasma Lp(a) level is above 30 mg/dL, the relative risk of CHD is raised about two-fold. When LDL and Lp(a) are both elevated, the relative risk is increased to about five-fold. A few ELISA assay methods for quantitating Lp(a) in plasma are known. ELISAs that are presently known use either monoclonal or affinity-purified polyclonal antibodies. Most of the monoclonal antibodies recognize the Kringle 4 epitope of apo(a), whereas the polyclonal antibodies recognize both Kringle 4 and Kringle 5 epitopes of apo(a). As noted above, apo(a) contains multiple copies of Kringle 4 domain. The multiple copies of apo(a) Kringle 4 are similar but not identical to each other and can be divided into 10 distinct Kringle types (Kringle 4 types 1 through 10). One copy each of Kringle 4 type 1 and types 3 through 10 is present per apo(a) molecule; Kringle

A Diagnostic Perspective on Heart Disease and Lipid Disorders

4 type 2, however, is present in a variable number of repeats (from 3 to >40) and are therefore responsible for the size heterogeneity of apo(a) and consequently Lp(a). From the structural sequence of Kringle 4 repeats it seems obvious that the immunoreactivity of the antibodies used in the immunoassays to measure Lp(a) concentrations will vary according to the number of epitopes available in Lp(a). Therefore, antibodies against apo(a) should be selected to be specific for that part of the apo(a) molecule that is independent of size polymorphism, i.e. for Kringle 4 domains other than type 2 or Kringle 5 domain.

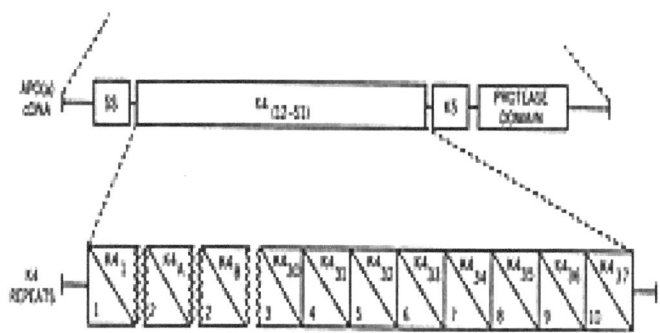

Structure of Lp(a)
(Taken from Samar Kundu US Patent No. 2001005134)

A Diagnostic Perspective on Heart Disease and Lipid Disorders

Most of the Lp(a) assay methods except the ELISAs are not commonly used known use either monoclonal or affinity-purified polyclonal antibodies. The majority of the monoclonal antibodies recognize the Kringle 4 epitope of apo(a), whereas the polyclonal antibodies recognize both Kringle 4 and Kringle 5 epitopes of apo(a). Among the numerous papers published to date, most of them Kringle 4 based antibodies which can cross react with plasminogen and can provide inaccurate results. Unfortunately, all commercial ELISA methods are variable and cannot be trusted.

As noted above, apo(a) contains multiple copies of Kringle 4 domain. The multiple copies of apo(a) Kringle 4 are similar but not identical to each other and can be divided into 10 distinct Kringle types (Kringle 4 types 1 through 10). One copy each of Kringle 4 type 1 and types 3 through 10 is present per apo(a) molecule; Kringle 4 type 2, however, is present in a variable number of repeats (from 3 to >40) and are therefore responsible for the size heterogeneity of apo(a) and consequently Lp(a) From the structural sequence of Kringle 4 repeats it seems obvious that the immunoreactivity of the antibodies used in the immunoassays to and are therefore responsible for the size heterogeneity of apo(a) and consequently Lp(a). From the

A Diagnostic Perspective on Heart Disease and Lipid Disorders

structural sequence of Kringle 4 repeats it seems obvious that the immunoreactivity of the antibodies used in the immunoassays to measure Lp(a) concentrations will vary according to the number of epitopes available in Lp(a). Therefore, antibodies against apo(a) should be selected to be specific for that part of the apo(a) molecule that is independent of size polymorphism, i.e. for Kringle 4 domains other than type 2 or Kringle 5 domain.

We have developed but not commercialized using these highly specific Kringle 5 monoclonal antibodies (obtained from Dr. Angeno Scanu of the University Chicago, IL) We have an (Samar Kundu: US Patent No. 2001005134) using these monoclonal antibodies specific for Kringle 5 of apo(a). An ELISA method was developed for directly measuring concentrations of Lp(a)] in a plasma sample. In one embodiment, the method involves the specific capture of Lp(a) from a plasma sample with a monoclonal antibody developed against Kringle 5 of apo(a), which is non-cross-reactive with plasminogen and Kringle 4 of apo(a). The quantity of the Lp(a) present in the sample is then measured by detecting the amount of Lp(a)-anti-Kringle 5 complex that has formed in the reaction. Alternatively, the Lp(a) may be captured non-specifically and then detected with the monoclonal antibody specific for Kringle 5 of apo(a). An

A Diagnostic Perspective on Heart Disease and Lipid Disorders

illustration of correlation between Lp(a)-Chol measured per our new procedure and widely use TERUMO ELISA is shown in Figure below. Similar correlation between TERUMO ELISA and the present method of using Sandwich ELISA with Kringle 5 as a capture antibody and Kringle 4 labeled with HRPO was seen with correlation coefficient R= 0.983 (Samar Kundu: US Patent US20010051347).

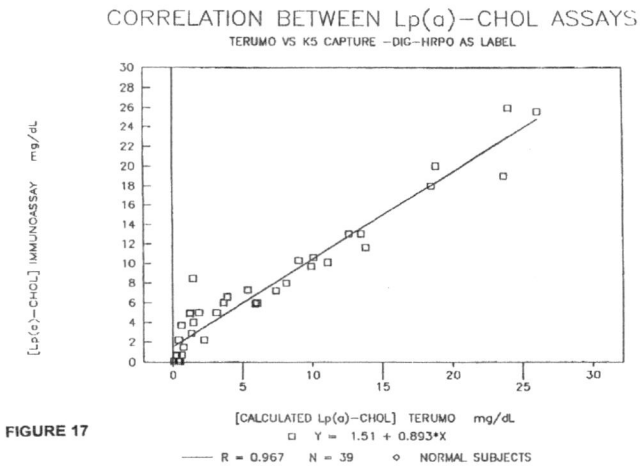

FIGURE 17

About 20% or one in five people have elevated levels of Lp(a) greater than 50 mg/dL from birth based on genetic factors they inherited from their parents, and most don't know they have it. Although high Lp(a) is a common condition, most people who are affected are undiagnosed. Approximately 30% of patients with FH (Familial

A Diagnostic Perspective on Heart Disease and Lipid Disorders

Hypercholesterolemia) have high Lp(a). Many doctors do not routinely test for it. The Lp(a) Foundation supports broader access to testing for Lp(a) levels for all people. And because it is inherited it is important to test all members of a family where one member is found to have high Lp(a) levels. It may only need to be tested once in a person's lifetime because it's genetic. Individuals with high concentrations of LDL- cholesterol and low HDL-cholesterol and family history of heart attack or stroke need to be tested for Lp(a). An estimated 50% of people who have heart attacks have normal levels of LDL-cholesterol.

The European Atherosclerosis Society (EAS) consensus panel recommended screening for elevated Lp(a), in people with moderate to high risk of cardiovascular disease. Desirable Lp(a) levels < 50 mg/dL were considered a treatment priority, after therapeutic management of LDL-cholesterol.

According to a statement from the EAS: ... *the evidence clearly supports Lp(a) as a priority for reducing cardiovascular risk, beyond that associated with LDL-cholesterol. Clinicians should consider screening statin-treated patients with recurrent heart disease, in addition to those considered at moderate to considerable risk of heart disease.*

A Diagnostic Perspective on Heart Disease and Lipid Disorders

b   Homocysteine

Homocysteine is a non-protein α-amino acid and a homologue of the amino acid cysteine. It is biosynthesized from methionine by the removal of its terminal C methyl group. Homocysteine can be recycled into methionine or converted into cysteine with the aid of certain B-vitamins. Homocysteine can be recycled into methionine or converted into cysteine with the aid of vitamins such as methylenetetrahydrofolate reductase, vitamin B6, and folate.

An elevated level of homocysteine in the blood (hyperhomocysteinemia) indicates that it is a significant risk factor for cardiovascular disease and makes a person more prone to endothelial cell injury leading to inflammation, atherogenesis and in ischemic injury. Hyperhomocysteinemia is therefore a possible risk factor for coronary artery disease. Its seriousness as a risk factor has been equated to hypercholesterolemia and smoking, two leading causes for cardiovascular disease. It also has been shown to produce a multiplicative effect with these and other risk factors such as hypertension. Two major hypotheses have been proposed to explain how homocysteine induces its harmful effects. It can damage endothelial cells lining the vasculature, allowing plaque formation. Simultaneously, it

A Diagnostic Perspective on Heart Disease and Lipid Disorders

interferes with the vasodilatory effect of endothelial derived nitric oxide. Also, homocysteine has been found to promote vascular smooth muscle cells hypertrophy. Maintaining a normal plasma level of homocysteine to prevent cardiovascular disease appears promising. This is achieved through increased intake of folate and vitamin B6 through diet or supplementation. Despite the overwhelming evidence suggesting homocysteine as a significant risk factor, no long-term prospective studies have been completed to demonstrate that folate and vitamin B6 can prevent cardiovascular disease related morbidity and mortality in patients with hyperhomocysteinemia.

Homocysteine levels are typically higher in men than women, and increase with age. Common levels are 10 to 12 µmol/L, and levels of 20 µmol/L are found in populations with low B-vitamin intake. The therapeutic targets for men are < 6.3 µmol/L and for women < 85 µg/dL

c. Heart-type (H-FABP) Fatty Acid-Binding Protein

Heart-type (H-FABP) Fatty Acid-Binding Protein Heart-type fatty acid binding protein (H-FABP) is a small soluble non-enzyme protein. It is one of the most abundant proteins in the heart and comprises 5–15% of the total cytosolic protein pool in the aqueous cytoplasm. H-FABP appears to be a

A Diagnostic Perspective on Heart Disease and Lipid Disorders

potential novel biochemical marker for the early diagnosis of myocardial infection. Under normal conditions, H-FABP is not present in plasma or interstitial fluid, but is released into the blood upon cardiac cellular injury. The cytoplasmic to vascular concentration of H-FABP is much higher in serum or plasma concentration of H-FABP under normal conditions which is < 5µg/L. This makes the plasma estimation of H-FABP a suitable indicator for the early detection and quantification of myocardial tissue injury.

Heart-type FABP is released into plasma within 2 hours after symptom onset and is reported to peak at about 4–6 hours and to return to normal base line level in 20 hours. A rise in serum and urine H-FABP concentration above reference values is seen in patients presenting with AMI as early as 1.5 hours after symptom onset. Serial measurements of H-FABP in the first 24 hours after onset of symptoms may be potentially useful for the diagnosis of AMI, to identify patients who need early reperfusion treatment and to detect re-infarction if it occurs early and for estimation of infarct size. However, some of the more recent studies have questioned the value of these early markers (H-FABP and myoglobin) when compared with specific markers like cTnI.

Heart-type FABP exists in high concentrations in the heart only. However, this protein is not totally cardiac specific and

A Diagnostic Perspective on Heart Disease and Lipid Disorders

occurs in other tissues although in much lower H-FABP is secreted by the kidney and circulates for a longer time (> 25 hours) after AMI in the presence of renal failure. Skeletal muscle damage during AMI may result in the leakage of H-FABP and an increase in Myoglobin concentration which could interfere with the results of the assays. The normal plasma concentration of H-FABP (< 5µg/L) is 10 to 15-fold lower than that of myoglobin (30–80µg/L). H-FABP is therefore more cardio-specific than myoglobin. These parameters, such as sensitivity, specificity, diagnostic efficacy and diagnostic accuracy, obtained for patients with chest pain within 3 hours and/or 6 hours after the onset of symptoms were almost the same as those for patients within 12 hours after symptoms. H-FABP is more sensitive than both myoglobin and CK-MB, more specific than myoglobin for detecting AMI within 12 hours after the onset of symptoms, and shows the highest values for both diagnostic efficacy and ROC curve analysis. Thus, H-FABP has excellent potential as an excellent biochemical cardiac marker for the diagnosis of AMI in the early phase. The plot below shows a comparison between F-FABP, Myoglobin, cTnI and CK-MB showing H-FABP as an earliest detector of AMI.

A Diagnostic Perspective on Heart Disease and Lipid Disorders

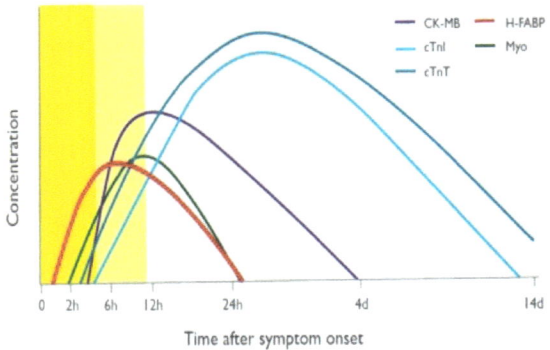

Detection of MI with F-FABP, Myoglobin, cTnI and CK-MB
(Source : https://quizlet.com/85209604/cardiac-biomarkers-flash-cards/)

d. Natriuretic Peptides: B-Type Natriuretic Peptide (BNP) and Amino Terminal- Pro B-Type Natriuretic Peptide (NT-proBNP)

Brain Natriuretic Peptide (BNP), also referred to as B-type natriuretic peptide. BNP represents the active hormone and when it is released from myocytes acts to reduce hemodynamic stressors such as wall stretch through natriuresis, vasodilation, inhibition of the renin-angiotensin-aldosterone axis and sympathetic nervous system. BNP has emerged as an important biomarker with an established role in the diagnosis of congestive heart failure (CHF). Investigators from several large studies examined the

A Diagnostic Perspective on Heart Disease and Lipid Disorders

performance characteristics of BNP testing in the acute care setting to assist in diagnosing CHF and in predicting long-term morbidity and mortality. Its utility has also been explored in myocardial ischemia and infarction, in right-sided heart failure (e.g., cor pulmonale), and in **acute pulmonary embolism** (PE). Furthermore, clinical trials are currently under way to determine if serial BNP measurements have a role in guiding the titration of CHF therapies.

Brain natriuretic peptide (BNP) is a member of a family of four human natriuretic peptides that share a common 17-peptide ring structure. The first was identified in 1983 and named atrial natriuretic peptide (ANP). ANP is a 28-amino acid polypeptide resulting from the C-terminal end of the prohormone proANP. The source is largely in the cardiac atria, and ANP is quickly secreted in response to atrial stretching. Normal hearts secrete extremely minimal amount of ANP, but elevated levels are found in patients with left ventricular (LV) hypertrophy and mitral valve disease. Before its activation, BNP is stored as a 108–amino acid polypeptide precursor, proBNP, in secretory granules in both ventricles and, to a lesser extent, in the atria. After proBNP is secreted in response to volume overload and resulting myocardial stretch, it is cleaved to

A Diagnostic Perspective on Heart Disease and Lipid Disorders

the 76-peptide, biologically inert N-terminal fragment NT-proBNP and the 32-peptide, biologically active hormone BNP. The 2 fragments are secreted into the plasma in equimolar amounts, and both have been clinically evaluated for use in the management of congestive heart failure (CHF).

High ventricular filling pressures stimulate the release of ANP and BNP. Both peptides have diuretic, natriuretic, and antihypertensive effects, which they exert by inhibiting the renin-angiotensin-aldosterone system. They also have systemic and renal sympathetic activity. In addition, BNP may provide a protective effect against the detrimental fibrosis and remodeling that occurs in progressive heart failure. Although ANP was identified first, concentrations of BNP in the myocardial tissue were found to be higher than those of ANP. Therefore, BNP has been studied more intensely than ANP as a clinically useful marker of increased ventricular filling pressure. An elevated BNP level is a marker of increased LV filling pressures and LV dysfunction.

NT-proBNP, on the other hand, is an inactive co-metabolite of the common intracellular precursor BNP and NT-proBNP are predominantly released from the cardiac ventricles in

A Diagnostic Perspective on Heart Disease and Lipid Disorders

response to hemodynamic stresses such as wall stretch or tension. Its utility has also been explored in myocardial ischemia and infarction, in right-sided heart failure, and in acute pulmonary embolism (PE).

Although BNP and NT-proBNP are most commonly associated with a clinical role in the diagnosis or rule-out of congestive heart failure, they have been evaluated for use in MI for prognostication, risk stratification, and rule-out of ACS in low-risk patients. Gene expression of this molecule is up-regulated in the presence of myocardial ischemia and thus a rational mechanism exists for its elevation in this setting, even in the absence of hemodynamic changes.

NT-proBNP's ability to indicate structural heart disease along with its correlation with ACS, infarct severity and prognostic implications post-MI confer the potential for its use in a variety of roles in the evaluation and management of this disease process. NT-proBNP's use in combination with cTnI has been shown in studies to improve the diagnostic ability of clinicians to differentiate between MI, unstable angina, and non-cardiac causes of chest pain. cTnI is the most heart-specific marker of myocardial damage, but NT-proBNP has been shown to have slightly better prognostic sensitivity. The incorporation of this marker into an algorithm to examine ACS reportedly adds to the

A Diagnostic Perspective on Heart Disease and Lipid Disorders

sensitivity of a single cTnI collection and allows for better negative predictive value. Although it is interesting, these data need to be confirmed before routine use is appropriate. In low risk patients, combining cTnI and NT-proBNP (or perhaps BNP) in a "rule-out" biomarker based model may provide the opportunity to safely discharge these patients without the current standard of care, stress test, saving the individual patient and healthcare system much aggravation and cost.

NT-proBNP has shown promise as a valuable marker of adverse outcomes in patients presenting with MI. In a large 70,000 patient's cohort presenting with MI, NT-proBNP was measured. Patient results were divided into quartiles, and there was a stepwise increase in in-hospital mortality from 1.3% in the lowest quartile to 11.2% in the highest quartile even after controlling for age, creatinine, heart failure, and shock]. A meta-analysis of 12 studies that included patients presenting to the hospital with NSTE ACS showed that risk of death was 4.89-fold greater in those patients with elevated NT-proBNP levels on admission.

The cardiac biomarkers cTnT, cTnI, BNP, and NT-proBNP provide valuable information for clinicians by assisting in the guidance of diagnostic, prognostic, and treatment decisions

A Diagnostic Perspective on Heart Disease and Lipid Disorders

for patients presenting urgently with signs and symptoms of MI. cTnT and cTnI have evolved through several assay revisions and currently the sensitive and high sensitivity versions of these assays are the best available tests for clinical use in MI diagnosis.

e. **C-Reactive Protein (CRP)**

C-Reactive Protein (CRP) is an annular (ring-shaped), pentameric protein found in blood plasma, whose levels rise in response to inflammation. It is known that an atherosclerotic process is characterized by a low-grade inflammation altering the endothelium of the coronary arteries and is associated with an increase level in markers of inflammation such as acute phase proteins and cytokines. Cumulative evidence indicates that inflammation, at both focal and systemic levels, plays a key role in destabilization and rupture of atherosclerotic plaques, leading to acute cardiovascular events. This suggests that inflammatory processes play a key role in determining plaque stability and biomarkers of inflammation may help to improve risk stratification and identify patient groups who might benefit

A Diagnostic Perspective on Heart Disease and Lipid Disorders

from treatment strategies. C-reactive protein (CRP), a prototype marker of the inflammatory process, is the most studied both as a causal factor and in the prediction of CHD.

CRP have been studied as noninvasive indicators of underlying atherosclerosis in apparently healthy individuals and of the risk of recurrent events in patients with established atherosclerotic vascular disease. However, the concentrations of CRP increase with age. Higher levels are found with viral and bacterial infections active inflammation, bacterial infection (40–200 mg/L), severe bacterial infections. Despite a lack of specificity for the cause of inflammation, data from more than 30 epidemiologic studies have shown a significant association between elevated serum or plasma concentrations of CRP and the prevalence of underlying atherosclerosis, the risk of recurrent cardiovascular events among patients with established disease, and the incidence of first cardiovascular events among individuals at risk for atherosclerosis. In addition, several drugs used in the treatment of cardiovascular disease reduce serum CRP. It is therefore possible that reduced inflammation contributes to the beneficial effects of these medications. In recent years, high sensitivity (hs) assay for CRP is commercially available.

A Diagnostic Perspective on Heart Disease and Lipid Disorders

The following is the CRP levels as determined by high sensitivity CRP assay:

- *low: hs-CRP level under 1.0 mg/L*
- *average: between 1.0 and 3.0 mg/L*
- *high: above 3.0 mg/L*

It should be noted that although CRP is associated with the inflammatory component of atherosclerosis, and an elevated CRP level has been linked with cardiovascular disease, based on the current available data it cannot be considered an independent risk factor for cardiovascular disease. The traditional risk factors for cardiovascular disease, including high blood pressure (hypertension), diabetes mellitus, elevated blood cholesterol, age, cigarette smoking, obesity, and family history of heart disease may correlate with an elevated CRP level. According to recent studies, after adjusting for these traditional risk factors, elevated CRP level alone is unlikely to be a cause of cardiovascular disease.

Nevertheless, CRP may be used as a predictor of cardiovascular disease based on its correlation with the other known cardiac risk factors and their role in the formation of atherosclerosis. In individuals with some of these traditional risk factors, the elevated CRP levels have been detected. Some data even suggest a trend of higher CRP elevation in the presence of higher number of risk factors.

e. **Myeloperoxidase**

Myeloperoxidase (MPO) is an enzyme, mainly released by activated neutrophils, characterized by powerful pro-oxidative and proinflammatory properties. Recently, MPO has been proposed as a useful risk marker and diagnostic tool in acute coronary syndromes Major evidence for MPO as enzymatic catalyst for oxidative modification of lipoproteins in the artery wall has been suggested in several studies performed with low-density lipoprotein. Recently, considerably interest is seen in MPO, that is abundant in ruptured plaque and can be measured in peripheral blood.

Recent studies suggest an association between elevated MPO levels and the severity of coronary artery disease (CAD). It has also been suggested that MPO plays a significant role in the development of the atherosclerotic lesion and rendering plaque unstable. MPO independently predicts CAD, and predicts a higher risk

A Diagnostic Perspective on Heart Disease and Lipid Disorders

of cardiovascular mortality, compared with patients with low MPO levels. MPO also improves risk model discrimination and patient risk category classification. It is interesting that elevations in multiple oxidative stress biomarkers predicts increased mortality risk; however, the strongest risk prediction can be achieved by assessing MPO and C-reactive protein (CRP) together. Patients with either MPO or CRP elevated had 5.3-fold higher cardiovascular mortality risk and patients with elevated levels of both MPO and CRP had a 4.3-fold risk compared with patients with only elevated marker. These results remained significant with adjustment for cardiovascular risk factors and baseline disease burden. Taken together, these data suggest that CRP and MPO may be complementary and explore different fields: CRP is a marker of disease activity and vascular inflammation, and is useful for long-term risk stratification while MPO is a marker of plaque instability and neutrophil activation and may be associated with short-term stratification, in patients with troponin negative level.

A Diagnostic Perspective on Heart Disease and Lipid Disorders

16. Conclusions

The purpose of this book is to put together a concise the present-day knowledge about Lipids and Lipid Disorders. It also covers Lipoproteins and associated diseases related to heart. It also emphasizes use of newer methods that would be beneficial in the diagnostic field. I intend to provide readers a perceptive of the cardiovascular biomarkers that are being used in the diagnosis, follow up, treatment and in future applications.

I have utilized the most modern-day scenarios from articles available in the website, additionally from Wikipedia Free Access for which I am highly obliged. I also acknowledge and thanks for the diagrams included in this book (which are free access or my own publications). Additionally, instead of providing an extensive list of bibliography, I included the most pertinent references for this book.

A Diagnostic Perspective on Heart Disease and Lipid Disorders

17. Bibliography

1. Cholesterol: https://en.wikipedia.org/wiki/Cholesterol
2. Triglyceride: https://en.wikipedia.org/wiki/Triglyceride
3. Phospholipid: https://en.wikipedia.org/wiki/Phospholipid
4. Hypercholesterolemia: https://en.wikipedia.org/wiki/Hypercholesterolemia
5. Lipid: https://en.wikipedia.org/wiki/Lipid
6. Cardiac Marker: https://en.wikipedia.org/wiki/Cardiac_marker
7. Sphingolipid: https://en.wikipedia.org/wiki/Sphingolipid
8. Sphingolipidoses: https://en.wikipedia.org/wiki/Sphingolipidoses
9. Lipid Storage Disorder: https://en.wikipedia.org/wiki/Lipid_storage_disorder
10. Farmingham Heart Study: https://en.wikipedia.org/wiki/Framingham_Heart_Study
11. Heart Failure: https://en.wikipedia.org/wiki/Heart_failure
12. C-Reactive Protein: https://en.wikipedia.org/wiki/C-reactive_protein

A Diagnostic Perspective on Heart Disease and Lipid Disorders

13. Lipoprotein(a):
    https://en.wikipedia.org/wiki/Lipoprotein(a)

14. Homocysteine:
    https://en.wikipedia.org/wiki/Homocysteine

15. Heart Fatty Acid Binding Protein (H-FABP):
    https://en.wikipedia.org/wiki/Heart_type_acid_binding_protein

16. Myeloperoxidase:
    https://en.wikipedia.org/wiki/Myeloperoxidase

17. A. M. Gotto, ed., Plasma Lipoproteins, Academic Press, New York, 1987

18. J. C. Fruchart and J. Shepherd eds., Human Plasma Lipoproteins, Walter DeGruyer, New York, 1989

19. Friedewald WT, Levy RI, Fredrickson DS. Estimation of the concentration of low-density lipoprotein cholesterol in plasma, without use of the preparative ultracentrifuge. Clin Chem. 1972;18(6):499–502.

20. Seth S. Martin, Michael J. Blaha, Mohamed B. Elshazly, Peter P. Toth, Peter O. Kwiterovich, Roger S. Blumenthal, and Steven R. Jones, Comparison of a Novel Method vs the Friedewald Equation for Estimating Low-Density Lipoprotein

Cholesterol Levels From the Standard Lipid Profile, JAMA. 2013 Nov 20; 310(19): 2061–2068.

21. Paul T. Williams, Xue-Qiao Zhao, Santica M. Marcovina, B. Greg Brown, Ronald M. Krauss, Levels of Cholesterol in Small LDL Particles Predict Atherosclerosis Progression and Incident CHD in the HDL-Atherosclerosis Treatment Study (HATS), Published: February 27, 2013 https://doi.org/10.1371/journal.pone.0056782

22. Eric H Yang, Lipid Management Guidelines in the Heart.org Medscape, 2015

23. Christie Ballantyne Bruce Arroll James Shepherd, Lipids and CVD management: towards a global consensus, European Heart Journal, Volume 26, pp. 2224–2231, 2005

24. Samar K. Kundu etal., Immunocapture assay for direct quantitation of specific lipoprotein cholesterol levels Patent No. WO 1993018067 A1, 1993

25. Samar K. Kundu etal, Immunoassay for detection of very low-density lipoprotein and antibodies useful therefor, US Patent 20030124743, 2003

26. Samar K Kundu etal., Specific antibodies to Kringle 5 of apo(a) methods of use therefor, US Patent 20010051347, 2001

27. Samar K. Kundu, Glycolipid Structure, Synthesis and Function, pages. 203-262, in "Glycoconjugates: Composition, Structure and Function", H. J. Allen and E.C. Kisailus, eds., Marcel Dekker Inc, New York, 1992

28. Robert Ledeen, eds., Ganglioside Structure, Function, and Biomedical Potential, Advances in Experimental Medicine and Biology, Springe, 1984

29. Thomas Kolter, Ganglioside Biochemistry Review Article, ISRN Biochemistry Volume 2012 (2012), Article ID 506160, 36 pages LDL Particle Number and Risk of Future Cardiovascular Disease in the Framingham Offspring Study – Implications for LDL Management

30. William C. Cromwell, James D. Otto's, Michelle J. Keyes, Michael J. Pembina, Lisa Sullivan, Ramachandran S. Vesna, Peter W.F. Wilson, and Ralph B. D Agostino LDL Particle Number and Risk of Future Cardiovascular Disease in the Framingham Offspring Study – Implications for LDL Management, Clin Lipidol. 1(6): 583–59, 2007

31. Ernst J Schaefer, Lipoproteins, nutrition, and heart disease1–6 Am J Clin Nutr 75: LDL Cholesterol and Other Lipids in Coronary Heart Disease

32. W P Castelli, J T Doyle, T Gordon, C G Hames, M C Hjortland, S B, HDL Cholesterol and Other Lipids in Coronary Heart Disease, The Cooperative Lipoprotein Phenotyping Study, Circulation 977;55:767-772, 2014

33. Eric Christenson, and Robert H. Christenson, The Role of Cardiac Biomarkers in the Diagnosis and Management of Patients Presenting with Suspected Acute Coronary Syndrome, Ann Lab Med; 33(5): 309–318, 2013

34. Donald Schreiber, Cardiac Markers in the Heart.org Medscape, 2017 emedicine.medscape.com/article/811905-overview

35. Ramachandran S. Vasan, Biomarkers of Cardiovascular Disease: Molecular Basis and Practical Considerations, Circulation, 113; 2335-2362, 2006

36. Amit Kumar Shrivastava, Harsh Vardhan Singh, Sanjeev Kumar Singh , C-reactive protein, inflammation and coronary heart disease, The Egyptian Heart Journal, 67, pp. 89-97, 2015

A Diagnostic Perspective on Heart Disease and Lipid Disorders

37. Hafidh A Al-Hadi and Keith A Fox Sultan Qaboos., Cardiac Markers in the Early Diagnosis and Management of Patients with Acute Coronary Syndrome, Univ Med J. 9(3): 231–246, 2009

38. Valentina Loria, Ilaria Dato, Francesca Graziani, and Luigi M. Biasucci, Myeloperoxidase: A New Biomarker of Inflammation in Ischemic Heart Disease and Acute Coronary Syndromes, Mediators Inflamm. 13562, 2008

39. Hafidh A Al-Hadi, Keith A Fox, Coronary Syndrome, SQU Med J, 9, pp. 231-246, 2009

40. Ravi Kant Upadhyay, Emerging Risk Biomarkers in Cardiovascular Diseases and Disorders, J of Lipids, Volume 2015 (2015), Article ID 971453, 50 pages

41. Sally P A McCormick, Lipoprotein(a): Biology and Clinical Importance, Clin. Biochem Rev 25(1): 69-80, 2004

A Diagnostic Perspective on
Heart Disease and Lipid Disorders

18. Dedication

I dedicate this book in memory of my

parents

Sushil Kumar Daskundu

and

Suprava Daskundu

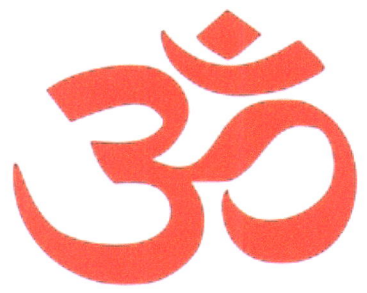

www.ingramcontent.com/pod-product-compliance
Lightning Source LLC
Chambersburg PA
CBHW040055250526
45473CB00041B/34

42. W.H. Wilson Tang etal, National Academy of Clinical Biochemistry Laboratory Medicine Practice Guidelines: Clinical Utilization of Cardiac Biomarker Testing in Heart Failure. Circulation: doi:10.1161/CIRCULATIONAHA.107.185267 2007;116: e99-e109; originally published online July 14, 2007; Circulation.

43. John R. Burnett, Lipids, Lipoproteins, Atherosclerosis and Cardiovascular Disease, Clin Biochem Rev, Vol 25 February 2004

44. Alan Chait and Robert H. Eckel, Lipids, Lipoproteins, and Cardiovascular Disease: Clinical Pharmacology Now and in the Future, J Clin Endocrinol Metab 101: 804–814, 2016

45. Kausik K Ray, Lipids and cardiovascular disease: re-thinking targets, Br. J Cardiol, 19 (Suppl 1): s1-s16, 2012

46. Wal Lee T. Wong etal., A Monoclonal-Antibody-Based Enzyme-Linked Immunosorbent Assay of Lipoprotein(a), CLIN. CHEM. 36/2, 192-197, 1990

A Diagnostic Perspective on Heart Disease and Lipid Disorders

47. Joseph L. Witztum and Daniel Steinberg, Role of Oxidized Low Density Lipoprotein in Atherogenesis, Clin. Invest 88, 1785-1792, 1991

48. Hanna Kim Gagging and James L. Januzzi Jr, Cardiac Biomarkers and Heart Failure An Expert Analysis, American College of Cardiology, February 2015